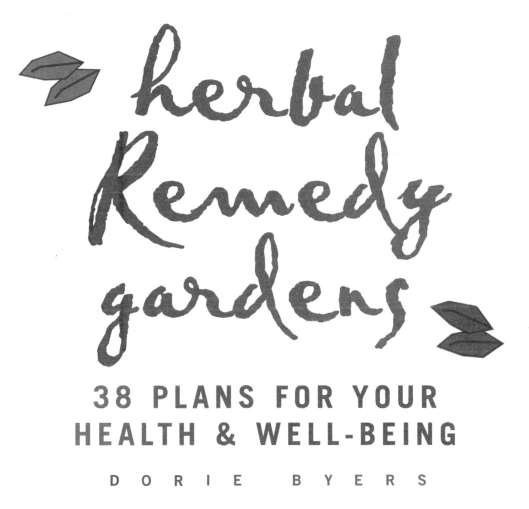

herbal Remedy gardens

38 PLANS FOR YOUR HEALTH & WELL-BEING

DORIE BYERS

STOREY BOOKS
Schoolhouse Road
Pownal, Vermont 05261

The mission of Storey Communications is to serve our customers
by publishing practical information that encourages personal independence
in harmony with the environment.

Edited by Deborah Balmuth and Robin Catalano
Cover and text design by Carol Jessop,
    Black Trout Design
Cover illustrations by Laura Tedeschi
Text production by Susan Bernier and Mary B. Minella
Garden plan illustrations in chapter 5 by Laura Tedeschi;
    all other illustrations by Beverly Duncan; except for
    pages 8, 22, 32, 52, 56, 58, 82, 83 (second), 164, 169
    (bottom), 171, 177, 194 (left), 195 (left) by Brigita
    Fuhrmann; pages 10, 30, 83 (first, fourth), 178 by
    Alison Kolesar; pages 18, 60, 196 (top) by Louise
    Riotte; pages 20, 26, 28, 40, 42, 44, 46, 50, 54, 169
    (top), 171 by Charles Joslin; page 166 by Judy Eliason;
    pages 184, 185 (first, third, fourth), 186 by Cathy
    Baker; pages 204, 207–210 by Regina Hughes
Professional assistance by Shatoiya de la Tour
Indexed by Hagerty & Holloway

The information in this book is true and complete to the
best of our knowledge. All recommendations are made without
guarantee on the part of the author or Storey Books. The
author and publisher disclaim any liability in connection with
the use of this information. For additional information, please
contact Storey Books, Schoolhouse Road, Pownal, Vermont
05261.

Storey books are available for special premium and pro-
motional uses and for customized editions. For further information, please call the Custom Publishing Department at
1-800-793-9396.

Printed in the United States by R.R. Donnelley
10 9 8 7 6 5 4 3 2 1

Library of Congress Cataloging-in-Publication Data

Byers, Dorie
    Herbal remedy gardens: 38 plans for your health & well-
being / Dorie Byers.
        p.   cm.
    Includes bibliographical references (p.   ) and index.
    ISBN 1-58017-095-1 (alk. paper)
    1. Herb gardening.   2. Herbs.   3. Herbs—
Therapeutic use.   I. Title.
SB351.H5B93   1999
615'.321—dc21   98-29971
                                               CIP

Contents

Acknowledgments

Writing a book involves far more than just putting words on paper. I want to give some credit to those who gave me assistance, inspiration, and encouragement.

First of all, I want to thank my husband, Rick, for being patient when I had to take time away from the home and family over and above the "workdays" I spent at the computer. He also gets an extra-special thanks for being available to help with the "keyboard crisis" when the manuscript was getting near completion. My thanks and love to you always.

As this book has grown and developed, so has our son, Jason. I hope that this book teaches him that anything is possible and that he should always follow his dreams. Thank you for your pride in my work and helping out when I was busy. I love you.

Also, thanks to Deborah Balmuth, Robin Catalano, and the rest of the staff at Storey Books for their assistance, hard work, and kind support.

The herb gardeners from all across the country who are featured throughout the book deserve a big thanks. They all took time out of their busy schedules to answer my questions so that their experiences and knowledge could be shared. It just reaffirms my belief that gardeners are some of the nicest people around. Many thanks.

Thanks to my sister-in-law Lauren Emme of Landscape Solutions in Glen Ellyn, Illinois, for all of the great gardening ideas. I hope that your gardening dreams continue to grow, Laurie!

Thanks to Sue for the gift of herb plants many years ago. Who would have thought that my interest in herbs would grow so much?

To Nancy Kirklin and her staff at Franklin Cornucopia in Franklin, Indiana, my thanks for giving me some insight into the herbal buying practices of their customers.

To Carol Chau, my friend since college, who surprised me with an unexpected phone call last winter. This led to a sharing of each others' newfound abilities and talents, which then evolved into Carol's gift of an herbal haiku. What better place to show off this gift than by opening a chapter of my book?

Additional thanks to Chuck Landon, DaHOM, DN, Ph.D., of Nature's Cupboard in Greenwood, Indiana, for some idea of the uses his customers find for herb preparations.

CHAPTER 1

An Introduction to Growing Medicinal Herbs

*H*ealing with plants is not a new idea by any means. For centuries, people have used plants from their own environments to heal, and to enhance their health. Many of these ideas, or "granny cures" as they have been called by many who now have revived their uses, were put aside in favor of more modern methods of healing early in the 20th century. Over the last two to three decades, healing with herbs has been rediscovered. This renaissance has come about with good reason, for modern research is affirming that many of the herbal treatments used through history by many cultures really do work.

If you like plants that are fragrant, practical, decorative, healing, tasty, nutritious, and otherwise useful, grow some herbs. The word *herb* can have different meanings for different people. To me it signifies any plant that can be put to cosmetic, culinary, decorative, aromatic, or medicinal use.

Gardeners who buy herbs, or receive them as gifts, often have questions about not only how to grow each herb, but how to use it as well. I find that most are eager for this knowledge, and pleased when they learn how versatile herbs can be. Many are surprised to find that certain herbs they had not thought of as medicinal can indeed have healing properties and promote general health. It is for this purpose that I am writing this book.

MULTIPLE-USE PLANTS

I have always been the type of gardener who wants to discover all of the uses of every plant I grow. And with herbs, multiple uses for each plant are definitely more the rule than the exception. Many of the plants that we use for food or decoration also have healthful qualities. Every time I discover yet another use for one of my herbs, I experience renewed excitement. I also continue to grow in my respect for these plants. To my way of thinking, they are some of nature's most useful gifts.

In this book I'll give you some ideas about using herbs in different ways and for different reasons than you may be accustomed to. The information comes from my own years of herbal discovery — reading about herbs and using them in a variety of ways. It is practical information that you can use to enhance your general health, and possibly relieve some self-limiting physical ailments. None of this information is intended to replace professional medical advice. Use it with moderation and common sense, though, and it can enhance your life and well-being.

I am happy to invite you along on my herbal journey. We all are on a road of discovery and there is much to learn — but I firmly believe that to learn is to grow.

THE BENEFITS OF HERB GARDENING

Growing herbs has given me great pleasure for many years. These plants often have pleasant aromas, and they're interesting and beautiful to look at. Gardening with them is a treat.

In spring, one of my first gardening tasks is to root out early grasses and weeds from my herb beds. This is not an unpleasant task, because even though weeding is not a lot of fun in itself, the herbs have so much sensory stimulation to offer me. I check the new plant growth that is peeking out, smelling and tasting when appropriate, and dividing any plants that need it. Most divisions get potted up to give to friends or to sell at garden club sales and my garage sales. To me, it is delightful that my herbs grow so abundantly that I can share them. And I love to imagine myself among these plants in another month or two, anticipating all that my family and I will do with them.

My spring interaction with herbs is not just confined to the outdoors. I also spend time checking my new herb plants under the grow lights in our guest-bedroom-turned-plant-nursery. I plant seeds early, frequently too early, because the cold, dark days of late winter make me eager to grow something new, and each seedling holds a promise of spring. Just seeing the new growth and smelling the aroma of these plants give me some relief from the gray, blustery weather.

Healing Effects

The act of gardening itself has many benefits; I believe it to be as therapeutic as any medicine. Its first advantage is exercise. If you've done any gardening, you're fully aware how much physical activity it can include. An added benefit is that you are outdoors and closer to nature; there is much to be learned by watching and listening while you are gardening. The birds always seem happy to keep a gardener company. The sky gives you different scenes, depending upon the clouds. The fresh air can act as a tonic to a mind weary from the tasks and worries of the day. I have read of gardening programs being offered in prisons to violent offenders; their violent tendencies lessened when they became involved. Knowing the immeasurable peace I've gained while gardening, I don't doubt this in the least.

A Place to Learn

A garden can teach you lessons of life, if you're willing to learn them. Gardening is the fostering of living things. There is nurturing involved, as well as observing how plants grow. You can't help but become a better person when you're taking care of plants.

Herbs have many culinary and medicinal uses, and are fun to grow.

Gardening is also an exercise in patience. You do not get immediate results from your efforts. Eventually, however, your garden will reward you with beauty and the bounty of a useful crop. These are well worth the time you waited.

Planning and growing various herb gardens offers you a flexible creative outlet. You can grow herbs in unconventional containers on a patio, or in rows or random groups on large plots of land. Herbs can be grouped according to their uses, colors, scents, or leaf textures. It is ultimately up to you.

PURSUING AN ANCIENT PASTIME

Herbs are as old as time. They have been used throughout written history, and most likely were used before that, too. When you grow and use them you are following in the footsteps of many generations before you, so you cannot study herbs without uncovering some of their history.

It is speculated that early humans discovered uses for wild plants through trial and error. When the hunter-gatherers settled down and became farmers, they cultivated the plants they'd found useful; these were the first crops. Anthropologists believe that as early as 7000 B.C., fatty oils of olive and sesame were combined with fragrant plants to create ointments. By the 28th century B.C., the Egyptians were writing about herbs in their papyrus manuscripts. The Sumerians followed with a written herbal record around 2500 B.C. By 700 B.C., traders in the markets of Athens were keeping written records of their heavy trade in marjoram, thyme, sage, and rose. About three hundred years later Hippocrates used many plants to treat diseases, which led him to become known as the father of medicine.

Medicinal uses of plants continued to be studied by the Greeks and other cultures throughout the next several centuries. Alexander the Great was asked by Aristotle to find out how other cultures were using the aloe plant. Alexander also sent plant cuttings from newfound varieties to a friend during his extensive travels. There are many mentions of herb use in both the Old and New Testaments of the Bible.

Written forms of herbal information waned during the Dark Ages, but monasteries nutured the written word and kept the ancient herbal manuscripts alive. The monks copied many writings, including herbal manuscripts, and kept gardens of herbs, usually planted near the dispensary so that the medicinal herbs were readily available for use.

During the next five hundred years new written records of herbal use appeared from time to time, by such diverse people as the Arab physician Avicenna (A.D. 980–1037) and Saint Hildegard the Abbess of Bingen (A.D. 1098–1179). By

A.D. 1300, Europeans were showing a renewed interest in herbs, using them in their households, in cosmetics, and as medicines. Another important application was strewing along the ground: When the herbs were walked upon, their fragrances were released, helping mask the odors of inadequate sewage disposal and unwashed bodies.

North American Migration

During the 1600s and 1700s, the European colonists of North America carried seeds of their most useful plants to the New World. The significance of this becomes clear when you consider that each colonist was allowed only limited cargo space and, in that space, seeds were given priority. Clearly, the colonists valued their plants highly. The herbs they introduced to their new land included plantain, mint, lavender, parsley, pot marigold (also known as calendula), roses, dandelion, chamomile, thyme, and yarrow.

Settlers planted their herb gardens just outside the doors of their new homes for convenience and safety. They also gained herbal knowledge from the Native Americans they met. The Arawak introduced Columbus and his crew to cayenne on the Canary islands. The Cherokee tribe showed the new settlers how to use goldenrod to treat fevers, and the Sioux showed western frontier settlers how to use echinacea to treat wounds and snakebites.

Thomas Jefferson, known primarily as a statesman and one of the founders of our country, was also a gardener who kept thorough records of his gardens at Monticello. Some of the herbs grown there were lemon balm, sage, mint, thyme, chamomile, rosemary, and lavender.

By the 20th century, the discovery of synthetic medicines caused the use of herbs as medicinals to fade. Interest did not revive on a large scale until the self-sufficiency movement of the 1960s. Now interest in using natural substances as alternative preservers of health and well-being has skyrocketed, making herbal knowledge more sought after than ever. Herbalists have been instrumental in helping along this revival by practicing and sharing their knowledge. Books and articles abound on their use of herbs, making the general population aware of the plants' abilities to heal and preserve health.

The Importance of Herbs

Herbs were extremely important in the times before clinics or hospitals. Doctors were not available to everyone then, either, and medications as we know them today were nonexistent. The common people used plant parts for treating different ailments,

---

HERBAL NAMES

When you are looking at herbs, check the Latin name of each plant. If the word *officinalis* is included, you can be sure that the herb was used at one time as a medicinal. *Officinalis* is a Latin word that means "of a storeroom," and indicates that the plant held enough importance to be kept for use should the need arise.

and dried the most useful herbs to store and use during the winter months. There was little formal research other than trial and error, with the results passed on by word of mouth. Printed herbals, texts which gave information on the use of herbs, for the general population were not available until the 17th century. It is interesting to me that recent herbal research has shown that many of these plants do indeed contain substances that aid in treating some of the same ailments. Our ancestors were on the right track!

WHY GROW HERBS?

Many grocery stores these days carry fresh herbs, and natural food stores sell bulk dried herbs. So you are probably wondering, "Why should I bother growing my own herbs?"

One reason is to be assured of the freshness of your herb supply. Those "fresh" herbs you find packaged in the produce department were picked an unknown time ago. How fresh are they really? When you go into your garden and cut some parsley, it doesn't languish on a shelf, losing freshness. Also, remember that buying any quantity of fresh herbs is much less economical than growing and harvesting your own supply as you need it.

When you buy fresh herbs, it's always possible that some have been exposed to natural and unnatural contaminants. Many purchased herbs are not available in an organic form. If you grow your own crop organically, though, you know that the pollutants affecting you have been minimized.

The same principle applies to dried herbs. Most bulk dried herbs are packaged in plastic bags, and have been exposed to air, light, and high temperatures for an unknown amount of time. All of these factors can cause them to lose their potency. But harvesting, drying, and storing your own gives you control over these processes.

I am not saying you must grow all of your herbs; that is not a practical notion. Even I can't grow all of the herbs I use. Do investigate your herb sources. Talk to some natural-food store owners about their choices for a reliable, safe supply of herbs. I find that many of these people try to maintain some kind of standard for the herbs they carry. Also, growing your own herbs will tell you what they smell and look like, and how they taste. This will become your "insurance policy" when you need to purchase bulk herbs: If it doesn't smell or taste like the herb you've come to know, then you probably aren't getting what you're paying for.

Growing herb plants from seeds can result in further savings to your pocketbook. For the price of one common herb plant at the nursery, you can buy a package of seeds and start many plants to use yourself, give away, or sell. You'll have the double bonus of saving the money *and* enjoying a fresh crop of herbs.

CAUTION: IMPORTED HERBS

Many herbs are imported from countries with less stringent standards of purity. When you purchase imported dried herbs, then, keep in mind that they may be adulterated with any number of substances, such as pesticides, insects, and other plants.

Additional Benefits

Growing your own herb plants can have another benefit: It can increase the populations of plants that are in danger of extinction because they are being destroyed and/or overharvested in the wild.

With herbs being used more often by increasing numbers of people, there are sure to be shortages in the years ahead. These can affect both the supplies of a plant you find useful, and the quality. As you become more practiced at growing herbs, you might want to try some that are being overharvested. These take a bit more patience to grow but are worth it for all who respect these plants' potential.

Almost anyone can grow herbs. You can cultivate them in great or small numbers, depending upon what space you have available. You don't need great amounts of acreage to grow herbs; small plots or containers can give you an adequate crop. Also, most herbs can adapt to many different climate and soil types.

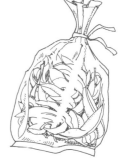

Bags of bulk herbs are sold in many health- and natural-food stores.

Choosing Which Herbs to Grow

Read through the descriptions of the herbs in this book and choose those that seem to suit your needs. Perhaps there are one or two in particular that will help you and your family enjoy better health.

Don't be afraid to grow an herb that is unfamiliar to you. I have discovered some herbs that I wouldn't do without by experimenting. Of course, some plants just won't thrive no matter what you do. Some may be invasive; you will have to dig them out. All this is part of the process of learning to grow herbs.

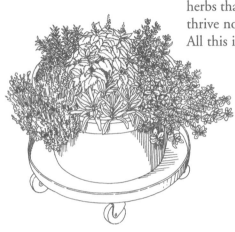

Containers are a great way to grow herbs indoors.

CHAPTER 2

Using Herbs as Medicine

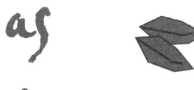

*H*erbs are a healthy addition to your life. They are very versatile, providing you with benefits such as enhanced nutrition, first-aid treatments, and remedies for minor illnesses. Self-treatment with herbs is inexpensive and a viable way to promote overall good health, but it's important to use them responsibly. Seek out a physician for diagnosis and consultation before you embark on an herbal regime. Keep yourself informed by reading and researching the most recent studies on herbal medicine. Do yourself and your physician a favor by sharing your findings: Give him or her copies of articles that are pertinent to you and your needs. New research is being done constantly on many herbs, and an ever-growing number of books is available, too. I recommend that you read several and use the information to help you form your own conclusions before you embark on any specific herbal treatments.

None of the herbs in these pages will give you a "miracle cure" for a disease or illness. They can, however, be supportive to you during times when your body is compromised, and can complement conventional medical treatments when indicated. Don't treat any pre-existing conditions with herbs before consulting your health professional. Be aware that some plants can cause allergic reactions. Also, there are specific parameters you must follow for treating children, the elderly, and pregnant women. Check your resources carefully for safety information before giving them any herbal treatments.

Finally, effects of herbs on ailments are usually quite gradual. These plants are not magic bullets or a quick fix. It takes patience, a proper attitude toward the plants, and an understanding of your body and physical condition to achieve the healing you desire.

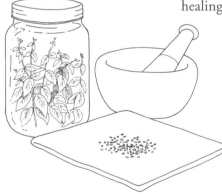

A mortar and pestle, jar, and towels are handy tools for processing and preserving your herbs.

MAKING HERBAL PREPARATIONS

The most common ways to prepare herbs to use for medicinal purposes are to brew them in hot water, or to prepare them in a base of oil or alcohol. You will find more specific recipes in Herbs to Know and Appreciate. The following are directions for different ways to prepare herbs.

Before using external herbal preparations, perform a patch test for possible skin reactions. Place a small amount of the substance on the inside of your forearm, and cover the spot with a bandage overnight. Remove the bandage in the morning. If no redness or irritation has occurred, the preparation should be safe to use on your skin.

Teas or Infusions

Teas (also called infusions) are a good way to get the benefits of an herb, and in some cases they can be a pleasant treat in your day, too. For best effect, use an infusion when you make it. It also can be stored in the refrigerator for 24 to 48 hours before discarding.

A Simple Tea

1. Place the specified amount of herbs (see individual recipes) in a heatproof container. If you don't want loose leaves in your tea, contain the herbs in a muslin tea bag, heat-sealable tea bag, or stainless-steel strainer or infuser.
2. Pour boiling water over the herbs.
3. Cover the container to allow the tea to steep for the prescribed amount of time, usually 15 to 20 minutes. The cover will keep the herbs' essential oils, which are quite volatile, from escaping.
4. Remove or strain the herbs from the infusion, and sip to enjoy.

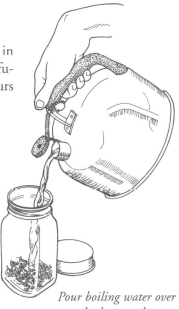

Pour boiling water over your herbs to make a tea or infusion.

Decoctions

Decoctions are infusions that are simmered to release the flavor, aroma, and active ingredients of the herb. This procedure is reserved for parts of an herb that do not release their culinary and/or medicinal properties as readily, such as seeds, roots, and bark. For best effect, use a decoction soon after you make it. If needed, you can store it for 24 to 48 hours in the refrigerator for later use, but you must discard it after that period of time.

A Basic Decoction

1. Crush the herbs with a mortar and pestle, or place them on a hard surface and strike with a wooden mallet.
2. Combine the herb and water in an enamel or stainless-steel saucepan. (See individual recipes for specific amounts.)
3. Simmer for the directed amount of time.
4. Strain or otherwise remove the herb from the liquid before using, then sip to enjoy.

Infused Oils

Herbal infused oils for external use can be made several ways. I always use olive oil, because its keeping qualities are superior to those of nut and other vegetable oils. Dried herbs are better than fresh, which have too high a moisture content and can cause the oil to grow mold or otherwise spoil. Herbal infused oils are for external use only.

Infused Oil—Method One

1. Combine 2 cups of olive oil and 1 cup of dried herbs in a slow cooker.
2. Heat on the lowest setting with the lid on for at least 4 to 6 hours, until the oil takes on the color and aroma of the herb.
3. Strain the infused oil into a dark glass bottle. Squeeze the liquid from two 400 IU vitamin E gelcaps into the infused oil to act as a natural preservative.
4. Label the bottle with its contents and date for storage.

Infused Oil—Method Two

1. Combine 2 cups of olive oil and 1 cup of dried herbs in a stainless-steel or enamel-coated pot.
2. Place the pot on the stove over low or medium-low heat. Watch carefully so that the olive oil does not burn or scorch.
4. Heat for 30 to 60 minutes until the oil takes on the color and aroma of the given herb.
5. Strain the oil and store it in a dark glass bottle. Squeeze the liquid from two 400 IU vitamin E gelcaps into the infused oil to enhance its keeping qualities.
6. Label the bottle for storage.

Infused Oil—Method Three

I find this the easiest way to make infused oil, as long as you are not in a hurry.

1. Place 1 cup of dried herbs in a clean glass jar with a snug-fitting lid. Cover the herbs with 2 cups of olive oil.
2. Place the jar inside a paper bag and set it in a sunny window. Let it sit for 1 to 2 weeks.

When making an infused oil, strain and store the liquid in a dark glass bottle.

3. Strain the herbs from the oil, reserving the oil. Add another 1 cup of dried herbs to the jar and cover with the reserved oil. Add a little more olive oil to cover the dried herbs if needed.
4. Leave the jar in a sunny window again for 1 to 2 weeks.
5. Strain the herbs from the oil, pouring the infused oil into a dark glass bottle.
6. Add the contents of two 400 IU gelcaps of vitamin E to the infused oil as a preservative. Label the bottle with its contents and date.

Tinctures

Tinctures are a simple and useful way to make the healing properties of herbs available to you. When prepared in an alcohol tincture, herbs can be kept for an indefinite period of time. To make a tincture, you need pure grain alcohol, also known as Everclear. If your state does not sell it, look for the highest-proof brand of vodka or brandy available.

Measure tinctures in drops according to the herb it contains and what you are using the tincture for. If you do not want to ingest the alcohol, place the drops of tincture in a small amount of warm water and stir. The alcohol will evaporate, leaving you with the herb.

Basic Tincture

1. Combine ¾ cup of alcohol with ¾ cup of distilled water in a jar with a tight-fitting lid.
2. Add 1½ ounces of dried herbs of your choice.
3. Replace the lid and place the jar in a cool, dark spot.
4. Shake the mixture daily for 2 weeks.
5. Strain the mixture to remove the herb. This must be done quickly or the alcohol will evaporate. I usually pour the mixture into a strainer lined with an unbleached paper coffee filter and place it in the refrigerator as it strains, to slow the evaporation of the alcohol. After straining, squeeze the filter to remove as much of the liquid as possible.
6. Store in a dark-colored glass bottle with an eyedropper fitted into the lid. Label the bottle, including type of tincture and the date.

CAUTIONS FOR USING HERBAL REMEDIES

- Always see a physician for serious physical ailments and diseases such as kidney disorders, heart disorders, high blood pressure, and any other chronic disorders.
- Always check that plants are safe to use to treat children, the elderly, or pregnant women.
- Make a positive identification of any plant before using it.
- Common names of herbs can vary from region to region. Be familiar with the Latin names of plants to be sure you have the right species.
- If after a week or two of herbal treatment, your condition has not improved, seek out the advice of your health-care professional.
- Start with the smallest possible amounts of herbs that will help you.
- Stop any herbal treatment if you are in doubt about plant identification, diagnosis of a physical condition, or the appropriate use of the treatment.

Herbal Salves

Herbal salves are made by melting an infused oil with an appropriate amount of beeswax to stiffen. This is also a good way to incorporate herbal essential oils into an application.

Basic Salve

1. Combine the specified amount (see individual recipes) of herbal infused oil and beeswax in a heat-resistant glass container.
2. Place the glass container in a pot containing 1 to 2 inches of water.
3. Bring the water to a boil and watch the ingredients carefully. Do not allow the pot to boil dry. When the contents of the glass container have melted and mixed together, remove the container from the boiling water.
4. Add the contents of two 400 IU gelcaps of vitamin E to the melted mixture to act as a natural preservative.
5. If herbal essential oils are called for in the recipe, add them to the melted mixture after it has cooled slightly but before it has solidified.
6. Store the salve in a low, widemouthed glass jar. Label the jar with its contents and the date it was made.

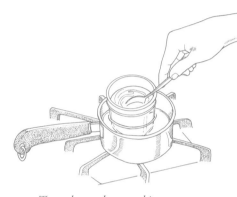

To make a salve, combine herbal infused oil and beeswax in a heat-resistant glass container and watch carefully while melting in boiling water.

STORING HERBAL PRODUCTS

Here are some hints on storage to help keep the results of your harvest and hard work at their optimal freshness and potency. Glass containers with tight-fitting lids are ideal for protecting the freshness of these products. Make sure that the containers are clean and completely dry before adding any herbal preparations. Dark-colored glass will help to keep light from degrading or breaking down your herbal products.

Label any containers of herbal preparations with the following information:

- the date the preparation was placed in the container
- the ingredients of the preparation, including the amount of each ingredient
- any specific instructions or cautions

Store herbal products in a place away from heat and direct light. A pantry or cupboard can be used, but avoid places such as cabinets above your stove. There could hardly be a worse place for storage, as the heat from cooking rises and quickly decreases the potency of your herbal products.

CHAPTER 3

Herbs to Know and Appreciate

his chapter contains descriptions of twenty-two herbs that I find useful for helping my family and me maintain optimal health. I grow each and every one of these herbs somewhere on our property. They have grown despite our unpredictable and often harsh midwestern winters, and the drought-ridden times of summer. (There is a saying in Indiana that if you don't like the weather, stick around and tomorrow it will change!) These plants have also grown despite some of my gardening mistakes, and occasional benign neglect. Many of the plants started out in my gardens as culinary or specimen herbs; it was only later that I discovered through reading and trials that they have other uses. A few of them, but very few, require some special care, although they are exceptions in my garden. Several, for instance, cannot survive our winters and must be moved into the house to live in containers. Still, I find that I get along best with plants I don't have to "baby"; if I repeatedly try to grow plants that don't like my soil or growing conditions, I surrender to their fussiness and omit them from my garden plans. Specific uses for each of these herbs can be found in Designing a Garden for Your Special Needs.

SELECTING PLANTS FOR YOUR REGION

Any of the plants in this chapter are good choices for a beginning herb garden. Keep in mind that some will require a trip inside for the winter in some areas; if you don't have the space or inclination to bring them in for the cold months consider them annuals. Check the growing zone requirements under each plant, then refer to the growing zone map for the herbs appropriate to your area. (See page 62.) Under the category "Will Grow in Zone," I have listed the growing zone or zones in which the plant will grow best followed by special information on the rest of the growing zones if there is any.

Do not become too fixated on growing-zone information. And by all means, do not limit your plantings if you find an herb that you want to plant but the growing-zone specifications do not include your area; it is not a cut-and-dried issue. Many plants that you purchase or raise from seeds and nurture will do well even if you do not live in a recommended growing zone. A lot of the success of growing herbs or other plants has to do with getting to know each plant and what it likes. Frequently you only will need to give the plant a special place in your garden, with shelter, partial shade, or a raised bed, for it to thrive in your location.

Different varieties of the same plant can have different medicinal properties. Other variables that affect plant properties can be uncontrollable conditions, such as weather, soil conditions, and pest or disease problems.

Start Small

If you are a new or seasoned gardener who is interested in starting herb gardening, begin with one or two herb plants. Take your time growing each plant, getting to know where they like to grow and how much space they claim. This will help you decide whether you like these plants, and if the plants prove useful for you and your family.

Make a list that includes the traits you desire in an herb plant. This list can include anything you like, such as plant hardiness and vigor, scent, blooms, medicinal usefulness, culinary usefulness, attractiveness, or lack of invasiveness. Using this list, take notes as you watch your newly introduced herbs grow. At the end of the growing season, evaluate your observations, and make conclusions about whether these are herbs you want as permanent residents in your garden.

Each growing season, add another new herb plant or two. Continue to evaluate the new plants.

Over the seasons, you will find herbs that you like — as well as a few that you don't. Some herb plants won't suit your climate, your garden, or your personal needs. Don't feel guilty about leaving them out of your garden plans; you'll still have many different herb plants to choose from.

I am living proof of this trial-and-error philosophy. After a little over a decade, and despite some plant failures, my herb gardens continue to grow and grow!

FOOD AS MEDICINE

As you read the suggestions for uses of these plants, note that I have included culinary ideas for many of them. This is not a new idea. For years, China has had health restaurants that serve special dishes devised to alleviate certain ailments and disorders. Likewise, the Japanese macrobiotic diet is intended to promote good health. Think of food as medicine. It is not an unreasonable concept and can be quite pleasant for you in the long run.

Charlemagne, the emperor of the Holy Roman Empire in the 9th century A.D., was an admirer of herbs. He even went so far as to decree what herbs should be raised in gardens throughout the land. He was thought to have said that herbs are "the friend of physicians and the pride of cooks."

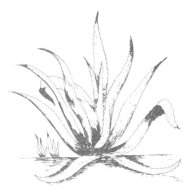

Aloe Vera *(Aloe barbadensis, A. arborescens)*

The aloe plant has been used on this planet for many centuries. Aristotle was thought to have asked Alexander the Great to investigate how other cultures used this plant. It is also believed that Alexander used aloe to help heal his troops during his African campaign. At times in history it was thought to provide protection and luck: To own an aloe plant was supposed to prevent household accidents.

Some believe that aloe prevents hair loss, although to my knowledge this use has never been proven effective. It has even been used for dental care. Ayurvedic physicians in India used aloe externally for burns, cuts, and traumatic wounds. Some research has shown that aloe vera gel can be effective in treating skin ulcerations. It has been found to accelerate wound healing and has some antibacterial and antifungal properties. An emollient and demulcent, aloe is a good choice for use in moisturizers and skin softeners.

ALOE GEL VERSUS ALOE JUICE

Do not confuse aloe vera juice with aloe vera gel; it is a different product altogether. The juice or latex is extracted from the green part of the leaf itself. Some people use this internally, and multiple health claims are made about it, but its use is not recommended because large doses can be cathartic.

Medicinal Uses

Suggested modern-day external uses of aloe gel include applying it to minor cuts, stings, bruises, blemishes, poison-ivy rashes, and eczema. My family and I use it for first-degree burn relief. I keep a plant within easy reach in my kitchen for first aid treatment of accidental cooking burns. We also apply it to any skin reddened by overexposure to the sun.

The gel should be applied topically. The fresher the gel, the better it works, which is why it is a good idea to keep a plant in your house. Fresh gel works far better than bottled commercial products. I have even seen bottles of aloe vera gel in stores that have been artificially colored blue or green!

Out of all the uses noted, providing first aid for first-degree burns seems to be the best use for aloe. In a first-degree burn, the skin is reddened, but without blisters or any other discoloration. To use the aloe gel, cut or break off a leaf, scrape out the gel, and apply to the affected area. Seek professional care if you suffer any burn that blisters, has evidence of destroyed tissue, or has been caused by electrical or chemical sources.

RAISING ALOE

Because of its cool green, succulent leaves, aloe has been commonly thought to belong to the cactus family, but in truth it is a member of the tree lily family. Most species originated in East and West Africa. In this country it is grown commercially in Texas, Florida, and southern California. If you live in a climate other than these, grow aloe in a container to bring inside when temperatures drop, because the plant will wilt and liquefy if exposed to temperatures below 40°F (4°C). For this reason, I classify it as a very tender perennial.

To grow, place in a container slightly larger than the plant with soil or planting mix that has good drainage. (The plant will survive in poor-quality soil, but it will not grow and thrive.) Water infrequently. Allow it to dry out between waterings. Some aloe plants tucked in windows in little-used rooms in my house have survived without water when I forgot about them for several weeks at a time. The aloe plant requires full sun to partial shade.

The plant will reproduce by forming little suckers, which are little shoots of new plant that originate from the roots. Once a year I remove the suckers from my mother plant, giving each sucker (which will have some small roots) its own container. Aloe reproduces so readily that you shouldn't have any trouble begging a start off someone who has a plant potted up on a windowsill.

If you live in a climate where the plant spends most of its time indoors, it probably will never flower. I have grown aloe plants for over 15 years, and never has one even hinted at flowering. What it lacks in bloom, however, it makes up for in usefulness. No one should be without one on their kitchen windowsill.

Growing at a Glance

Optimal Growing Conditions:
Warm, dry
Will Grow in Zone: 9 to 10;
in other zones you must container-grow aloe as a houseplant
Common Propagation:
Division of suckers
Type of Plant:
Tender perennial
Used in: First-Aid Garden (page 108), Traveler's Herb Garden (page 148), and Windowsill Medicine Cabinet (page 160)

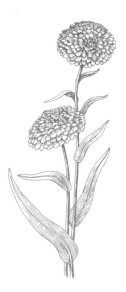

Calendula *(Calendula officinalis)*

Whenever I give an herb talk or class, a fair number of people are surprised when I bring out my jar of dried calendula blossoms. Most people don't think of calendula as an herb; they view it as a colorful annual. The name *Calendula* comes from the Latin word *calends,* meaning "the first day of the month," probably signifying the long amount of time this plant stays in bloom.

The length of bloom, however, is only one of calendula's advantages. The plant is a symbol for protection. It was used to elicit psychic powers and prophetic dreams among some groups of ancient people. A wealthy older Parisian circa 1390 wrote to his young wife that calendula was used to draw "evil humors" from the head. In the 17th century in Europe, it was used to cure plague and pestilence. It was one of the herbs that colonists brought with them to North America, most likely for culinary and healing purposes. The leaves of the plant were used on open wounds by battlefield doctors during the American Civil War.

Medicinal Uses

Known in the past as pot marigold because of its culinary uses, calendula has been around for centuries. Ancient Egyptians thought of it as a rejuvenating herb. Indian, Arabic, and Greek practitioners of medicine have long used calendula for its antiseptic and wound-healing properties. Calendula is related to the ragweed family, so do not use it if you have such allergies.

Recent studies in Germany found calendula to be effective in the reduction of inflammation and the promotion of healing in wounds. In addition, various studies have shown that calendula has antifungal, antiseptic, astringent, and anti-inflammatory properties. Once again, modern research has substantiated an ancient medicinal use of an herb. I find it quite interesting when this substantiation occurs, for it proves that through trial and error our ancestors found valid uses of the herbs available to them.

USING CALENDULA INFUSIONS

Use an infusion of calendula petals as a mouthwash and gargle for sore mouths. Additionally, you can use the infusion on sunburned skin and to clean cuts and scrapes. Gauze pads soaked in the infusion are helpful as eye compresses for tired, irritated eyes. Calendula infused oil is helpful to irritated skin and can be used to make calendula salve, a good substance to use on rashes, minor cuts, scrapes, and insect bites.

In addition, the edible bright orange or yellow petals contain beta-carotene, a precursor to vitamin A. These petals were used as a saffron substitute for many years and can still be seen today sprinkled fresh in salads or baked into cookies.

RAISING CALENDULA

Growing calendula is fairly easy. Into warm, well-worked soil, sow the seeds and barely cover them. The plant prefers well-drained, rich soil, but it will grow in much poorer growing conditions. With minimal care, it will reward you with lots of brightly colored blooms. For a new crop of calendula next season, allow a few blooms to go to seed, sprinkling the seeds over the bed to distribute them more evenly if you desire. If not, transplant the new seedlings and move them to other places in spring when they are 3 to 4 inches tall.

For a head start, calendula seeds can be started early in containers before transplanting into the garden. I tend to have better luck transplanting seedlings into the garden than sowing seeds directly into the ground. The plant is tolerant of a wide variety of weather conditions, although it does best in cool to moderate temperatures.

There are several varieties of calendula available, ranging in height from dwarf varieties 6 inches tall to others as tall as 1 to 2 feet. Pick the variety that best fits into your landscape.

Harvesting

To harvest, pick in the afternoon when the blooms are newly opened. The more blooms you pick, the more you will encourage the plants to bloom again. After drying the blooms, remove the petals and store them. This is the part of the plant that contains the active constituents.

Growing at a Glance

Optimal Growing Conditions: Warm soil; tolerates a variety of soil conditions
Will Grow in Zone: 3 to 10; in Zones 8 to 10, it must be treated as a cool-weather annual
Common Propagation: Plant seeds — it will reseed itself
Type of Plant: Annual
Used in: Bath Garden (page 88), Eye Care Garden (page 104), First-Aid Garden (page 108), Hair Care Garden (page 112), Skin Care Garden (page 136)

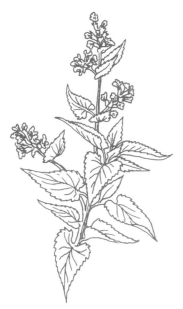

Catnip *(Nepeta cataria)*

Several years ago, I was showing a neighbor around my yard and gardens. When we got to the catnip, she started to smile. "When we were little," she said, "my mother always gave us catnip tea when we were sick."

A member of the mint family, this Mediterranean native was once thought to symbolize love, beauty, and happiness. In pre-Elizabethan England, people drank catnip tea in the afternoons. Gardens in colonial America included catnip plantings.

Medicinal Uses

Commonly thought of as a treat for cats and frequently found stuffed in cat toys, this useful herb can also promote rest, improve digestion, calm and soothe stomach upsets, and relieve the symptoms of colds, flu, and fevers. It even contains antiseptic properties with which minor skin lesions can be treated. The volatile oils contained in catnip can absorb intestinal gas, so it is an age-old remedy for childhood colic. Taken before meals, it can be used to stimulate the appetite. The fresh leaves contain vitamins A, B, and C.

Catnip's ability to help you relax and sleep has been compared to valerian's. It is calming without being disruptive of the next day's activities. For an aid to rest, use 1 to 2 teaspoons of dried herb per cup boiling water. Cover the cup to keep the volatile oils from evaporating and let the infusion steep for 15 to 20 minutes, then strain. Use the same infusion to alleviate cold and flu symptoms, and to help settle a stomach upset from indigestion and/or gas.

Cautions

As you can see, catnip's uses are many and varied. From the catnip-stuffed toys found in pet stores to memories of teas prepared by mothers in days gone by, catnip can be a useful addition to your medicine chest. However, you should not use catnip if you are pregnant.

RAISING CATNIP

Raising catnip is easy. My first and only patch of catnip was grown from a free packet of seeds scratched into the heavy clay soil on the western side of our corrugated metal shed. There it grows year after year, spreading out some but not as drastically as its mint cousins are apt to do. It will also self-seed. The seeds germinate best when they are shallowly planted. Further propagation can be accomplished by dividing mature plants or by cuttings.

CATNIP FOR CHILDREN

Catnip will help soothe a colicky stomach and relax a child who has a cold and fever. For children and toddlers, give only 2 teaspoons of the cooled infusion. (A hot infusion can burn the mouth or tongue.)

The plants will thrive in well-worked, rich soil and they enjoy moderate moisture, but during dry spells I rarely water my plants and they survive. They like full sun but tolerate partial shade. The 2- to 3-foot-tall plants have gray-green leaves and clusters of white fuzzy-looking blooms on top, which honeybees love. The plants are said to deter flea beetles, although I have never experimented with this.

To harvest, dry the leaves on their stems before the plants bloom. Strip the leaves from the stems to store. Do not crumble the leaves until you are ready to use them.

"Cat Proofing" Your Catnip

Atypically, my cats do not roll around and make a mess of the catnip patch. I have heard of people who had to put little wire cages around their catnip so that they would have some to harvest, because their cats go wild in it. Old folk wisdom says if you plant catnip from seeds the cats won't notice it, but if you transplant plants they will notice it immediately and love it to death. Perhaps that is why my catnip goes unscathed. Only my cats know the real truth of the matter, and they're not telling.

If you have a problem with feline friends destroying your catnip crop, plant plastic forks with the tines up around and in your catnip bed. The fork tines will poke at your cats when they try to roll in the bed; this should deter them. In extreme cases, fashion a chicken-wire cage over the catnip. If you are feeling particularly generous, and you have the space to spare, plant a separate patch of catnip away from the rest of your garden for your cats. There they can roll around to their heart's content without destroying your crop, or any other plants that have the misfortune of being in proximity to the catnip.

Growing at a Glance

Optimal Growing Conditions: Adaptable to a variety of soil types, likes warm temperatures

Will Grow in Zone: 3 to 10; the plants may winterkill in Zones 3 and 4

Common Propagation: Seeds, division, cuttings (will reseed itself readily)

Type of Plant: Perennial

Used in: Children's Herb Garden (page 92), Cold and Flu Garden (page 96), Decongestant Garden (page 100), and Tummy Care Garden (page 152)

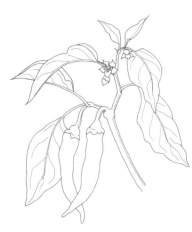

Cayenne Pepper *(Capsicum annuum)*

Grown in India, Africa, and the New World, cayenne was brought to Europe by Christopher Columbus. It was used in food preparation, and was specifically used in Africa to induce skin-cooling sweats, no doubt quite welcome in the African climate. The plant symbolized fidelity to some.

Columbus would have been disappointed to learn that in the 17th century, European herbalists believed cayenne emitted dangerous vapors. It's not hard to see where this opinion came from, though: If someone unfamiliar with the herb takes a close whiff, it will result in reddened, watery eyes and a sharp intake of breath.

Medicinal Uses

Despite such misgivings about cayenne, its uses are many. It enhances circulation, helping hot conditions cool off and cold conditions warm up. When used topically it is a counterirritant, bringing blood to the surface of the skin and causing reddening. As such, it is used to help relieve the pain of arthritic joints. Cayenne promotes digestion, increases appetite, promotes sweating, and is stimulating and energizing. Nutritionally it contains vitamins A, C, and E. It is also a natural antioxidant.

Cayenne's active ingredient is capsaicin. The hotter the pepper, the more capsaicin it contains. A low concentration of capsaicin in topical creams for muscle and joint aches and pains has been available commercially the last few years. Consistent topical use for four or five times a day for at least 4 weeks seems to block pain pathways to affected areas.

Additional research is being done on using cayenne to treat cluster headaches. I doubt we are fully aware of all this plant's uses.

Aside from the topical application, eating cayenne is the best way to reap its benefits. Regularly including cayenne in your diet is supposed to enhance your circulation and improve digestion. It will also clear up sinus congestion. Some people have heartburn when eating cayenne — start by adding a pinch at a time and increase the amounts to suit your palate and your stomach. The negative effects of cayenne on the digestive system can be counteracted by eating a high-protein, low-fat diet.

Cautions

Always use caution when handling cayenne. Wear gloves when preparing it, and keep it away from your eyes. Do not apply cayenne to damaged skin. Cayenne is not recommended for people with active ulcers, and ingesting large amounts of this herb

WARM YOURSELF WITH CAYENNE

For colds and chills, place ¼ to ½ teaspoon dried cayenne in 1 pint tomato juice and warm the mixture, stirring until the cayenne is distributed. Sip ½ to 1 cup at a time for a heat-producing, sinus-clearing, vitamin-packed drink. Store the remainder in the refrigerator for later use and rewarm before drinking.

For adults only, sprinkle ½ to 1 teaspoon ground cayenne pepper in your socks on cold days when you are going to be outside. This will help your feet to feel nice and warm.

can be harmful to the digestive tract and, possibly, kidneys. To decrease the heat of cayenne in your mouth, eat some rice or bread or drink milk; water only spreads the oil around. To remove cayenne residue from your skin, use a rinse of vinegar or milk.

RAISING CAYENNE

Cayenne loves heat and full sun. One summer we toured horticultural gardens divided by glass domes into different climates. In the "desert" climate grew pepper plants, which obviously liked it there, because they were 3 or 4 feet tall and loaded with fruit. Cayenne is even tolerant of dry conditions. In the heat of summer, when the rest of your plants are wilting, the cayenne pepper plants will still be going strong.

I like to start my pepper plants in early spring for a strong plant to move outside in late spring. Presprouting seeds seems to work the best for me. To presprout, place the seeds in a single layer on a damp paper towel, roll up the paper towel, and place it in a resealable plastic bag. You can put this on top of the hot-water heater, heat register, or any place consistently warm. Check the seeds after a couple of days and every day thereafter. When they have started to sprout, plant them shallowly in containers with damp, sterile potting mix. Place in a warm spot that receives 16 hours of strong light a day.

Transplant cayenne plants into your garden after all danger of frost is past. These heat lovers would never survive a frost. The plants themselves will grow into 2- to 3-foot-tall and 3-foot-diameter "bushes" with 3- to 6-inch-long slender slightly curved fruits that are green and turn red when ripe. The redder the fruits, the higher their vitamin content.

Harvesting and Storage

To harvest, pick the ripe red fruits while leaving the stem on. String the fruits on heavy string or fishing line, piercing the stems only, and hang this in a warm place out of direct sun until dry.

After they are dry, you can store the peppers whole or grind them into powder in your food processor. Use care when doing this, for pepper dust in the air can be quite irritating. Do not remove the cover from your food processor until all of the dust has settled. Store dried cayenne pepper in a glass jar away from heat and light.

Growing at a Glance

Optimal Growing Conditions: Warm to hot soil and air temperatures
Will Grow in Zone: 5 to 10 with lots of sun and heat; cayenne is hardy in Zone 10
Common Propagation: Seeds, transplants
Type of Plant: Annual
Used in: Cold and Flu Garden (page 96), Decongestant Garden (page 100), Healthy Heart Garden (page 120), and Rejuvenation Garden (page 128)

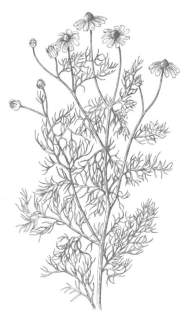

German Chamomile *(Matricaria recutita)*

Whenever I give a class to children, or even adults, I mention the end of the story *Peter Rabbit* by Beatrix Potter. Peter's mother was quite wise and gave Peter spoonfuls of chamomile tea to calm Peter down and help him rest after his difficult day.

Peter Rabbit's mother wasn't the only one to use chamomile for its healing properties. The Anglo-Saxons looked to chamomile as one of the nine sacred herbs given to heal the world by the god Odin. The early Egyptians and Romans used it to cure illnesses, too. Additionally, it was thought to bring love and money to the user.

Medicinal Uses

Chamomile will not only help you rest and calm down, but it has antispasmodic, carminative, analgesic, antiseptic, anti-inflammatory, and vulnerary properties as well. It's no wonder that it is famous for relieving such a wide range of ailments.

Chamomile's active ingredients are found in its volatile oils. These oils are also what give chamomile its fruity apple fragrance, which is so distinctive that in Central and South America chamomile is known as *manzanilla* or "little apple."

I once attended a talk by a well-known herbal expert and author, who was asked what herbs he liked to use. He replied that whenever his stomach was upset, he drank a cup of chamomile tea. The volatile oils of chamomile do help to soothe the lining of the gastrointestinal tract. When drunk between meals on an empty stomach, chamomile tea can help reduce flatulence. It also has the ability to cleanse and tone the digestive tract.

Chamomile is related to ragweed, asters, and chrysanthemums. If you have allergies to any of these plants, avoid using chamomile. Also, excessive use of chamomile tea can cause vomiting.

USES FOR A CHAMOMILE INFUSION

- Mouthwash for a sore, inflamed mouth.
- Lotion to soothe itchy skin, and skin reddened from the sun or wind.
- After-shampoo hair rinse to provide shine to hair.
- Tea to help relax yourself to sleep after a stressful day.

Chamomile doesn't affect consciousness, but will calm your nerves so that you may sleep.
Note: Store leftover infusion in the refrigerator and discard after 2 days.

There are two common kinds of chamomile. Roman chamomile or *Anthemis nobilis* is different in several ways from German chamomile. It is a low-growing perennial that can be started from seeds or plant divisions. It is antiemetic, antispasmodic, and mildly sedative. It promotes digestion and increases appetite. The flowers are what's used, just as in German chamomile. If you're in doubt about which is which, split open the yellow middle of the flower from the top of the flower to the stem. If it is hollow, it is German chamomile. If it is solid, it is Roman chamomile. *Note:* Do not use Roman chamomile if you are pregnant.

RAISING CHAMOMILE

Chamomile is so easy to grow that anyone can do it. This herb is forgiving of all soil types, and you can simply scratch its minuscule seeds lightly onto the top of the soil. Do not cover the seeds. In a week or two tiny, feathery seedlings will emerge. The plants will grow to about 1 foot tall with feathery foliage and have ¾-inch-diameter blooms that look like little daisies with bright yellow centers. The blooms appear in succession over a 2- to 3-week period, then the plant will gradually stop blooming and dry out as the summer weather gets hotter.

Plant early in the growing season. The seeds will germinate at 55°F (13°C). The plants themselves will grow in moist (not wet) or dry conditions. If you let a few of the flowers dry on the plant, it will reseed itself easily. I haven't planted any chamomile seed for years — the plants keep growing in the same spot due to reseeding. You might even have some plants in places where you didn't expect them. I always use the excuse that the garden fairies put them there.

Harvesting

Harvest the flowers just when they open, and dry thoroughly to prevent mold from forming. The flowers should be gathered daily. When you have a small patch of chamomile to harvest, it doesn't take long to gather the flowers; if you grow a larger quantity, though, try a harvesting "rake," which is similar to those used in blueberry harvests. You will need two dozen or more plants to reap an appreciable chamomile crop, but if you plant a whole packet of seeds you shouldn't have any trouble growing that many plants.

Growing at a Glance

Optimal Growing Conditions: Cool to warm, well-worked soil

Will Grow in Zone: 4 to 10; in zones with hot summers, it is grown as a cool-weather annual. Can possibly grow in Zone 3.

Common Propagation: Seeds; self-seeds readily

Type of Plant: Annual

Used in: Bath Garden (page 88), Children's Herb Garden (page 92), Eye Care Garden (page 104), Hair Care Garden (page 112), Headache Relief Garden (page 116), Relaxation Garden (page 132), Skin Care Garden (page 136), Traveler's Herb Garden (page 148), Tummy Care Garden (page 152), and Woman's Care Garden (page 156)

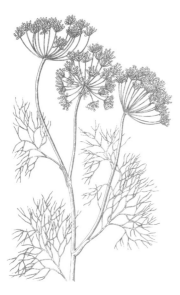

Dill *(Anethum graveolens)*

When giving seminars, I always ask children if they have ever eaten herbs. Typically, they will answer no. Then I ask if anyone has been to a hamburger place in the last week or two. Invariably most of the hands in the room go up and I then use the example of a dill pickle to illustrate that herbs have indeed been in their diets.

Fragrant dill is a useful and tasty herb with a long and interesting history. The plant is said to have originated in the Mediterranean. The Greeks and the Romans burned dill seeds as incense. The Romans also chewed the seeds to promote digestion, and the Egyptians used them for the relief of gas. In the Bible the book of Matthew mentions dill being used as a tithe. The Romans found dill so useful that they took it with them all over Europe and planted it wherever they settled. Its usefulness continued into the Middle Ages when, besides its more common applications, it was believed to prevent storms. In some cultures, dill was thought to symbolize protection, money, lust, and love. European colonists brought dill to this country, where they chewed the seeds during church services.

Medicinal Uses

Dill is one of those herbs that gives you two different crops — something I believe makes it even more desirable to grow. The finely cut green foliage is a flavorful seasoning either fresh or dried. It is also useful in herb blends to help decrease your salt intake. The seeds likewise give a distinctive flavor to different foods, as well as being a helpful aid to digestion.

Dill seeds relax the smooth muscles of the digestive tract and help prevent gas bubbles from forming in the intestines. For this reason, dill makes a useful addition to your medicine cabinet. To use, make a dill-seed infusion. Dill seeds will freshen your breath if you chew a few seeds. This is for adults only — the seeds are too small for children and could cause choking.

DILL SEED INFUSION

This infusion has long been a wonderful treatment for stomach and intestinal cramping due to gas (also known as colic) in babies. Add 2 teaspoons bruised dill seeds to 1 cup of water, simmer for 15 minutes, then strain. Adults may take 2 to 4 tablespoons at a time, and babies and small children may have 2 teaspoons of the cooled infusion at a time.

Another surprise is the nutritional content of dill seeds. One tablespoon of seeds contains 100 mg of the mineral calcium — more than you'll find in ⅓ cup of skim milk. Consequently, dill seeds make a healthful addition to your diet from a nutritional standpoint.

RAISING DILL

Dill is another easy-to-start, self-seeding annual that will give you a perpetual crop. Plant the seeds somewhere you would like to keep your dill year after year. Dill prefers a well-worked soil, because it has a taproot. Starting in early spring, scratch the seeds into the soil. They need light to germinate, so don't cover the seeds. In a week or so you will see little feathery seedlings that, with care, will grow to 2- to 3-foot-tall plants that are about 6 inches wide.

Harvest the foliage by snipping it off the sides of the stems. The plants will eventually have yellow umbel flowers that will attract beneficial insects; from these the small brown seeds will form. Allow a few of the plants (one or two is plenty) to drop their seeds onto the ground, where they will sprout and grow again.

For containers, choose a deep (8 inches or deeper) container to accommodate the taproot. Due to this taproot dill doesn't transplant very well, so starting the seeds ahead of the season for moving out into the garden isn't a good idea. It isn't really necessary anyway, since the seeds will sprout in the ground in early spring, and the plants will likely be ready for harvest before your first cucumbers.

For a succession of fresh dill, plant a crop every 2 weeks throughout the growing season. Do not plant near fennel, because this will cross-pollinate with it.

Butterflies are attracted to the dill flowers. I have even seen their colorful caterpillars feeding on dill foliage. Don't kill these "baby" butterflies. They will eventually reward you with the beautiful adult creatures.

Harvesting

To harvest foliage, continually snip it and dry by the usual methods. To harvest seeds, watch the umbels and, when the seeds are starting to fall, cut the stems 6 to 8 inches below the umbels and place them upside down in a paper bag. Tie the paper bag shut with a string, bundling up the stems along with the top of the bag, punch a few small holes at the top, and hang it up to dry. The seeds will fall into the bag as they dry; you can then easily collect them for storage.

Growing at a Glance

Optimal Growing Conditions: Cool to warm soil, full sun

Will Grow in Zone: 3 to 10; in Zone 8 and further south, treat dill as a cool-weather annual

Common Propagation: Seeds; reseeds readily

Type of Plant: Annual

Used in: Children's Herb Garden (page 92), Mouth Care Garden (page 124), and Tummy Care Garden (page 152)

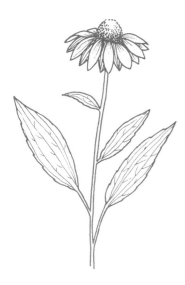

Echinacea *(Echinacea purpurea, E. angustifolia)*

Commonly known as the purple coneflower, the name *echinacea* seems to be on everyone's lips these days, and it is certainly in print everywhere. Best known for their ability to boost the immune system, echinacea pills fill the shelves of health-food stores as well as drugstores. The plant is well known not only by people familiar with herbs but also by those who aren't usually in the "herbal know."

Medicinal Uses

Native Americans taught the European settlers how to use echinacea. They had been using the plant to treat snakebites, fevers, wounds, and poisonous insect bites for a long time. In the 1880s in the United States, a pharmaceutical manufacturer started to sell different forms of echinacea. By the 1920s it was the country's most popular medicinal plant, but it lost favor when new and effective synthetic medicines appeared.

The German Commission E, a special committee of their Federal Department of Health, reviews the effects of herbs and their safety and publishes the results. It has approved echinacea for combating recurring infections, and local application for treatment of hard-to-heal wounds. This latter use has been justified by studies that show an accelerated healing rate of bacterial skin infections when echinacea is applied.

The plant's other properties include antiseptic, antimicrobial, lymphatic, and tonic. Usually, echinacea's root is the part used, although the aerial part of the plant has been used successfully in some preparations.

By and large echinacea is best known for and most widely used to stimulate and/or support the body's immune system against bacterial and viral attacks. At the first sign of cold or flu, start taking echinacea. Take doses of echinacea during waking hours for two days, then stop. Check the labels of your echinacea preparations for correct dosages. A general guide is 30–60 drops of echinacea tincture 3–6 times a day, or 2–5 size 0 capsules 3–6 times a day. It is not meant to be taken on a regular basis, only as an immune-system booster when needed. *E. purpurea* will not cure a cold or flu if you take it after the illness has taken hold.

Cautions

Echinacea can cause adverse reactions in people who are allergic to sunflowers. Do not use echinacea if you have a severe systemic immune disorder such as multiple sclerosis, tuberculosis, or a collagen disease such as lupus or scleroderma. Echinacea should be used with caution by pregnant women.

RAISING ECHINACEA

Growing your own echinacea is a good idea, since it is being harvested to extinction in the wild. Very little effort is needed to grow echinacea. The seeds do need to be stratified. I put the seeds into damp vermiculite and place in a recloseable plastic bag. Then I put the bag in the refrigerator for a month. After that time, I plant the seeds in flats and place under grow lights in a warm place. In less than a week, my seeds will have sprouted. When the weather outside has settled and danger of frost has passed, transplant the seedlings outside. The plants will grow slowly at first. Expect no flowers the first year.

If you want flowers the first year, mature echinacea plants can be divided and transplanted. They are available from local nurseries and by mail order. Echinacea multiplies readily and most neighbor gardeners will willingly give you a division.

Echinacea prefers a sunny location. It is even happy on the southern side of my house right next to the brick, which soaks up a lot of heat in the summer. It grows to about 3 feet in height and will spread gradually as far as you let it.

The petals of the flowers are a mauve color with orange-brown centers. When the plant blooms, expect a wonderful show of butterflies. When the blooms are finished, they will dry out and reseed themselves in your flower and herb beds; remove the spent blooms if you don't want this to occur.

Harvesting

To harvest echinacea, dig the roots after the plant has bloomed — usually in early fall. Only harvest 2- to 4-year-old roots, making sure that you leave enough plants for future use and propagation. Wash and dry the roots thoroughly, then chop them coarsely. Store the dried roots in a tightly covered glass container and keep away from direct heat and light.

> ## Growing at a Glance
>
> **Optimal Growing Conditions:**
> Full sun, warm to hot soil
> **Will Grow in Zone:** 3 to 9
> **Common Propagation:**
> Seeds, division
> **Type of Plant:** Perennial
> **Used in:** Cold and Flu
> Garden (page 96) and
> Traveler's Herb Garden
> (page 148)

USING ECHINACEA TINCTURE

Echinacea's active ingredients aren't all water soluble; a tincture is the best way to obtain its benefits. Use the instructions on page 13 to make a tincture using chopped root.

At the first sign of cold or flu's onset, many herbal experts recommend 30 drops of tincture every 3 hours for the first 2 days only. Once you have developed a full-blown case of a cold or flu, echinacea probably will not cure it.

If you are unable to take the alcohol in the tincture, add the tincture to a small glass of warm water and stir gently. The warm water will cause the alcohol to evaporate.

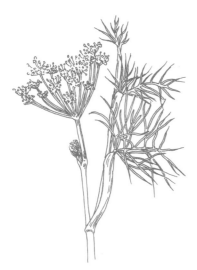

Fennel *(Foeniculum vulgare)*

This tall (approximately 4–6 feet), feathery-leafed plant has been appreciated for many centuries. Early Greeks called it *marathon,* supposedly after the city of Marathon, where fennel was said to grow in profusion. The Mesopotamians used it as a carminative. The Emperor Charlemagne had it planted on his imperial farms. In medieval times, fennel was one of nine sacred herbs believed to have the power to cure certain diseases. The plant symbolizes protection, healing, and purification. Today, most of us know fennel as the seeds used to season Italian sausage.

Medicinal Uses

It is the seeds of this plant that make it a most useful addition to any medicinal garden. The properties claimed for fennel are as a carminative, aromatic, antispasmodic, stimulant, galactogogue, rubefacient, and expectorant. Active ingredients in the seeds seem to be contained in their volatile oils.

Fennel's use as a digestive-tract treatment is probably its best known. Infusions of fennel seeds can help relieve flatulence and colic by absorbing intestinal gas. The plant can aid in calming upset stomachs, soothe an irritated gastrointestinal tract lining, and aid digestion. It is also known as an appetite stimulant. This is contradictory to the belief that fennel can be used to promote weight loss, an idea probably brought about by the fact that the seeds have a mild diuretic (water-expelling) effect.

An infusion is the best way to take fennel. Crush 1 to 2 teaspoons of the seeds and place in 1 cup of boiling water. Cover and let steep for 10 minutes, then strain and use. This infusion is not meant to be taken excessively or over a long period of time. An occasional cup is appropriate, but prolonged use can be irritating to several of the body's systems due to the volatile oils it contains.

An infusion of fennel seeds will help promote the flow of breast milk in nursing mothers. The infusion's volatile oils are passed on to the nursing infant via the breast milk. This will help to allay any digestive upsets in the infant.

Fennel's leaves and stems contain calcium, iron, potassium, and vitamins A and C. This plant part is familiar in cooking, particularly in seafood dishes. The flavor of the foliage is lost in the drying process. Use it fresh or not at all.

Cautions

There are some precautions to mention when using fennel. The first is that pregnant women should avoid ingesting fennel in anything but a normal culinary recipe, because

FENNEL'S COSMETIC USES

An infusion of fennel can be used as a cleansing lotion for the skin. It is best for mature skin; mix it with clay, yogurt, and/or wheat germ for a face mask. The circulatory stimulation effect of fennel brings blood to the skin's surface and will aid in softening the skin. Be sure to do a patch test first. You can also chew a few of the seeds as a breath freshener.

the herb is a uterine stimulant. The second precaution is to be very careful about harvesting fennel in the wild: It is easy to confuse with poison hemlock.

RAISING FENNEL

Fennel seeds are fall-planted and kept moist for early-spring germination here in the Midwest. The seeds prefer rich, well-worked soil. Plant the seeds at the back of your beds due to the height of the mature plants. Their height may also require that you stake or support the plants in some way. Fennel can have a tough time surviving winter in some places; its hardiness is not consistent. Try it in more than one place in your garden and see where it does best.

The umbel flowers of fennel attract beneficial insects as well as butterflies. If left unharvested, fennel will self-seed new seedlings. Leave some to replace old woody plants. Mature fennel plants can also be divided.

An interesting color variation can be found in bronze fennel, a different variety than the common one. The unusual-colored foliage can make a unique visual focal point or contrast in your herb garden.

Harvesting

After seeds form and begin to turn brown on the umbels, harvest by cutting the stems 6 to 8 inches long. Place the heads into a paper sack, tying it shut around the stems. As the seeds dry, they will fall into the sack. Store them in a glass container away from direct heat and light. You can snip the feathery foliage from the plant as needed.

Finally, do not confuse perennial fennel with the annual bulbed fennel. When harvested, the annual form can be cooked and used as a vegetable.

Growing at a Glance

Optimal Growing Conditions: Full sun, rich moist soil
Will Grow in Zone: 3 to 10; in far northern growing zones the plants may not mature enough to produce seeds
Common Propagation: Seeds, division
Type of Plant: Perennial
Used in: Children's Herb Garden (page 92), Mouth Care Garden (page 124), Tummy Care Garden (page 152), and Woman's Care Garden (page 156)

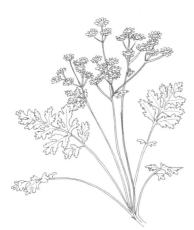

Feverfew *(Chrysanthemum parthenium)*

Despite its name, feverfew has never been documented to cure fevers. Its name is thought to be a corruption of *featherfew,* used to describe the white petals of the plant's small daisylike flowers. It is thought that the Romans were the first to start taking this herb for headaches. They also mixed feverfew with honey and sweet wine to alleviate vertigo and melancholy. The Greeks used it to aid contractions allowing the woman to deliver the placenta at childbirth.

Medicinal Uses

Feverfew seemed to fall out of favor in the Middle Ages and has been back in the spotlight only in the last few years, due to a British study. This study suggested that feverfew is useful in reducing the frequency and severity of migraine headaches.

Another study in the works concerns using the herb to treat acute arthritis attacks. The study was initiated when it was discovered that some British people self-medicate with feverfew because in doing so, they experience a decrease in the severity of their arthritis attacks.

Feverfew is vasodilatory, relaxant, and a uterine stimulant. The active ingredient in the feverfew plant appears to come from the plant's leaves and is called parthenolide. The amount of this ingredient can vary from plant to plant; thus, so can feverfew's effectiveness. If you want to use your own feverfew, harvest the leaves before the plant flowers and use them fresh or freeze them for later use. It has been recommended by various sources that one fresh or frozen leaf be eaten one to three times a day.

Cautions

Feverfew leaves are bitter tasting. Drinking an infusion is most unpalatable and not recommended. Do not take feverfew if you are taking anticoagulants, commonly known as blood thinners, and do not take if you are pregnant. People with a sensitivity to feverfew can develop mouth ulcers when eating the leaves. To prevent this, eat the leaves between two small pieces of bread.

STORAGE TIP

To provide a source of feverfew year-round, take clean, dry feverfew leaves and freeze them individually on a cookie sheet. Once frozen, remove them from the sheet and store in recloseable plastic bag. Remove leaves one at a time to use as needed.

RAISING FEVERFEW

Feverfew is a pretty plant. The lacy leaves and small white-petaled, daisylike flowers are a visual treat in flower beds. The cut flowers look nice in arrangements. Bees, however, don't like the plant.

Sow the tiny seeds directly into well-worked soil early in spring. Don't cover the seeds with much soil — just scratch them in. Feverfew prefers rich soil but shows no fussiness when planted in clay soils. In a short time, you will have hordes of tiny little lace-leafed seedlings. Usually they come up so thickly, due to the number of seeds, that you will want to thin them out. You can even transplant some of them when they grow to be 2 to 3 inches tall. The plants will thrive in full sun but will also do moderately well in partial shade. The mature plants can grow to about 2 feet tall. Harvesting leaves can encourage bushiness.

The plants bloom in early summer. After blooming, I usually cut off the drying flowers and discard them because feverfew will self-seed all over the garden if the flowers are left to dry on the plant. I have plants growing in places that I know for a fact feverfew never touched. I guess I'll have to blame these on the garden fairies!

Here in Indiana, feverfew plants that grow in sheltered spots are practically evergreen. If yours succumb to cold weather, they will be among the first plants to green up and grow come spring. If you yearn to grow things after the dreariness of late winter, feverfew is a welcome plant to add to your garden plans.

Growing at a Glance

Optimal Growing Conditions: Full sun, rich soil
Will Grow in Zone: 5 to 10; in Zones 8 to 10, treat feverfew as a short-lived annual
Common Propagation: Seeds
Type of Plant: Perennial
Used in: Headache Relief Garden (page 116)

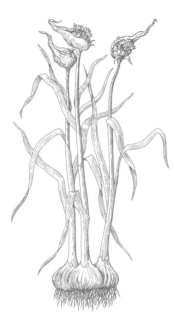

Garlic *(Allium sativum)*

Because the plant has been around for millennia, it is difficult to know where to start when discussing garlic. It's one of the oldest-known cultivated plants. The Egyptians believed that it prevented illness and increased strength and endurance. It is even rumored that the workers who built the pyramids ate garlic to sustain them in their labors. Greek athletes ate garlic before participating in races, and Greek soldiers ate garlic before battle. When the Romans conquered Gaul, they brought garlic with them. Nowadays garlic, also known as the "stinking rose," is believed to help alleviate many ailments. It's also said to symbolize protection and healing. Perhaps that is why, in folklore, it is said that wearing a garland of garlic will protect you from vampires.

Medicinal Uses

Garlic's properties include antiseptic, antiviral, diaphoretic, cholagogue, hypotensive, and antispasmodic. It has sulfur-containing compounds, enzymes, B vitamins, minerals, and flavonoids. In its raw form garlic can act on bacteria, viruses, and alimentary parasites. For this reason it can be used as a preventive in many infectious conditions. The volatile oils that give garlic its scent are excreted by the lungs and through the skin.

The best news on garlic seems to be on its effect on the cardiovascular system. Studies have suggested that, with regular use, garlic helps reduce blood cholesterol levels and blood pressure. This has helped to make garlic a best-seller in the vitamin and supplement world today. To lower cholesterol, you must eat the equivalent of two cloves a day.

Other positive studies imply that garlic may help AIDS patients by increasing killer-cell activity and possibly inhibiting malignant cell formation. The downside to all of this news is that garlic can cause heartburn in susceptible people. Additionally, its odor is offensive to some individuals. (If you're concerned about odor, there are deodorized garlic preparations available.)

The best way to take garlic is by eating it. Cooking garlic destroys its antibacterial and antiviral properties; it must be eaten raw to achieve those purposes. Cutting or crushing the cloves before eating them increases their effectiveness. There are many wonderful recipes that include this flavorful bulb. Cutting or crushing the cloves before eating them allows garlic to be more effective, because its active ingredients are released readily into your system. If you are concerned about your breath, chew some fresh parsley after eating garlic.

Cautions

Garlic can thin the blood. Avoid using it if you are already taking blood thinners or are planning to have surgery in the near future. Excessive topical use of this herb can cause irritation. The use of garlic other than in culinary amounts during pregnancy and nursing is not recommended.

RAISING GARLIC

There are two types of garlic that you can grow, depending on your location. Softneck varieties are the most productive; these are the ones found in grocery stores. They like mild winters and store very well. This is the garlic that is most commonly seen braided. Hardneck types like cold winters and are the best choice for areas that have changing seasons.

I find garlic trickier to grow than I expected. After separating the cloves from the bulb, you must plant them 2 inches deep into rich, well-worked soil. This is important: If your soil is heavy clay and/or stripped of its nutrients, you will end up with a harvest of tiny garlic bulbs. Cloves are best planted in fall 6 weeks before the ground freezes to allow root formation. After the first freeze, mulch the site to protect the soil from heaving and evicting the bulbs from their growing place.

In spring after the weather has settled, remove the mulch. Your garlic cloves should be sprouting green foliage that is wider and more strappy than that of onions. The plants will grow throughout summer. During the first month or two, they will appreciate a good watering once a week from you if nature doesn't provide it.

Harvesting

Near the end of summer or early fall, bend the tops over to encourage drying. When the tops start to shrivel, harvest the bulbs. Don't let them get too brown; this is a sign that the bulbs are rotting. Cure, or dry, the bulbs under hot, dry conditions. After they are cured you may cut the stems, or braid the garlic if you're feeling creative.

The bulbs will store best in cool (not cold), dry conditions. I have found that the small ceramic storage pots with holes in the top that are specially designed for garlic (available at kitchen supply stores) provide great storage conditions at room temperature.

Growing at a Glance

Optimal Growing Conditions: Rich soil, long growing season
Will Grow in Zone: 5 to 10; hardneck varieties can possibly grow in Zones 3 and 4
Common Propagation: Cloves
Type of Plant: Annual
Used in: Cold and Flu Garden (page 96), Healthy Heart Garden (page 120), and Rejuvenation Garden (page 128)

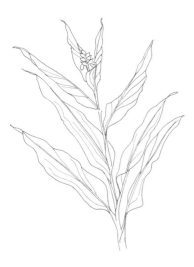

Ginger *(Zingiber officinale)*

In the United States, ginger is commonly thought of as a baking spice. For the last few years, though, the fresh root has also been available in Asian dishes, giving them a warm to hot, distinctively spicy flavor. I have come to enjoy this tropical rhizome so much that I keep it on hand to use and have even started growing it.

Ginger was brought to Europe via the trade routes from the Far East. Four to five thousand years ago, the Greeks were importing ginger. The herb was prominent in Chinese herbals circa 3000 B.C., and in India ginger has been widely used in Ayurvedic medicine. Spanish conquistadors brought the herb to the New World via Jamaica. To different cultures ginger has been said to symbolize love, money, success, and power.

Medicinal Uses

Nowadays, fresh ginger is becoming more popular in our country. It is rich in volatile oils whose properties include stimulant, antispasmodic, anti-inflammatory, carminative, rubefacient, and diaphoretic. The spicy rhizome also contains powerful antioxidant properties.

Ginger's actions on the digestive tract are notable. It works indirectly to increase the availability of dietary nutrients for digestion and metabolism. It promotes the gastric secretions that aid in digestion of food. Ginger is also a gastrointestinal tract stimulant. While it will aid in relieving nausea and indigestion from various causes, it can also reduce the nausea associated with motion sickness; some studies have found ginger to be superior to pharmacological substances in this. Take ginger at the first sign of queasiness when traveling for it to be effective.

Ginger is also stimulating to the peripheral circulation, making it a good topically applied treatment for minor muscle aches and pains. It relaxes peripheral blood vessels, bringing blood to the skin's surface and causing a counterirritant effect.

Taken as a tea, ginger can help to alleviate cold and flu discomfort, including sinus congestion. For feverish conditions, it can promote perspiration. Although culinary use during pregnancy is all right, larger quantities of ginger during pregnancy are not recommended.

Cautions

Avoid excessive intake if you suffer from peptic ulcers. Ginger may raise blood pressure, so avoid it if you have high blood pressure. Ginger may increase the activities of blood-thinning drugs.

GINGER TEA

This tea is fragrant and flavorful. It is a very pleasant way to take action against an upset tummy.

1 teaspoon fresh ginger, grated
1 cup boiling water
1 lemon slice
½ teaspoon honey, or to taste

Place the ginger in the boiling water. Let it steep, covered, for 15 minutes. Strain and cool to lukewarm. Add a thin lemon slice and a very small taste of honey for sweetness. Sip the infusion slowly.

RAISING GINGER

The first time I planted a ginger rhizome was the middle of winter, and the plant struggled to grow in the dry, slightly cool atmosphere of my house. When warm weather came I put the pot outside in a partially shaded area; when it got hot and we received lots of rain, the rhizome sprouted a multitude of leafy green stalks.

True to its nature as a tropical plant, ginger enjoys heat and moisture. To grow ginger, buy a firm ginger rhizome (also known as gingerroot) at the grocery store. Avoid the rhizomes that are shriveled and/or moldy. Have a container 10 to 12 inches wide prepared with a potting mixture that facilitates good drainage. Place the rhizome about 1 inch deep into the mix. You can place the rhizome with its flat side parallel to the top of the potting mixture, or perpendicular to the bottom of the container. It seems to grow equally well either way.

Place the container in a warm, partially shady situation and keep the soil continuously moist. I like to fill the dish the container is sitting in with water, and refill this as the moisture is taken up by the contents of the container. Be patient — the rhizomes take quite some time to sprout. Put the container outside in the warm months, taking care to provide continuous moisture and partial shade. You will be rewarded with a thriving tropical plant after a few weeks. Ginger will even bloom given the right conditions. I have not been fortunate enough to achieve this, although I have heard of it.

Harvesting

To harvest, dig up the rhizome no earlier than 9 weeks after it started growing, cut or break off what you need, and replant what is left. Peeled fresh ginger can be used chopped up or grated. The root can be wrapped and frozen for future use.

Growing at a Glance

Optimal Growing Conditions: Hot, moist

Will Grow in Zone: 9 to 10; in growing zones farther north, you must container-grow ginger and take it inside with the onset of cold weather

Common Propagation: Rhizomes

Type of Plant: Tender perennial

Used in: Children's Herb Garden (page 92), Decongestant Garden (page 100), Sore Muscle Care Garden (page 140), Traveler's Herb Garden (page 148), Tummy Care Garden (page 152), and Windowsill Medicine Cabinet (page 160)

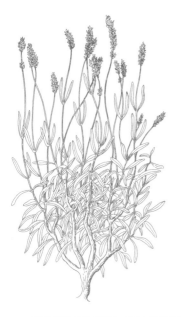

Lavender *(Lavandula* spp.*)*

Used since Roman times as a perfume, lavender has made a fragrant return to herb lovers everywhere. In the Middle Ages, it was thought to be the herb that symbolized love. A contradictory belief held that if lavender water was sprinkled on your head it made you chaste.

It came to England from southern France and became indispensable there for its clean, distinctive fragrance. Lavender was stuffed into skullcaps in 16th-century England and worn as a headache cure. Herb beds in colonial America were planted with lavender. During the early 1900s and during World War I, lavender was used as a wound disinfectant. The herb represents love, protection, sleep, chastity, purification, happiness, and peace.

Medicinal Uses

Lavender's properties are as an aromatic, nervine, carminative, stimulant, and tonic. The scent of lavender will assist someone in need of a tension reliever and calming influence. For this reason, lavender is an appropriate and popular ingredient in bath mixtures and little herb-stuffed "pillows" upon which you rest your head while going to sleep. The scent is also refreshing and deodorizing. It is often recommended to help lift the spirits. Some people use it to relieve headaches. Whether there is a scientific basis for this claim remains to be seen, but perhaps the aroma of the lavender is pleasing enough to help relieve the stress or tension associated with the headache.

Lavender is a good herb for practically all skin types. The infusion can be used as a fragrant rinse as well as for a skin-toning lotion. An infusion of lavender buds contains tannins, which help to relieve the discomfort of a sunburn. Use the infusion as a lotion over affected areas of the skin. Lavender may also be eaten in small amounts. It adds a distinctive aromatic flavor to sugar cookies.

As with all herbs, use lavender in moderation. Although the use of lavender seems relatively safe, a small percentage of the population might be allergic to this herb.

USING LAVENDER INFUSED OIL

Follow the directions for infused oil outlined on page 12, using lavender buds as your herb of choice. Use the fragrant rose-colored oil as a sore muscle rub, or add to an herbal salve recipe instead of regular oil to receive the benefits of lavender in topical applications.

RAISING LAVENDER

For years I yearned for a line of bushy flowering lavender plants in my herb beds. I would regularly go out each spring and buy a variety of lavenders, plant them — and then watch them all wither, dry up, and die. I wasted so much money on lavender, but I didn't stop trying to grow it. Finally, a couple of years ago, a variety called "Lady" lavender was introduced and I now have the beautiful bushy lavender plants I once dreamed about. This variety readily starts from seeds and reliably blooms the first year you plant it. "Munstead" lavender grows reliably from seed as well, but it will not bloom the first year.

All other varieties must be propagated by cuttings, because they do not grow reliably from seeds. There are many to choose from, including Spanish lavender *(L. stoechas)*, which will thrive in southern climates as a tender perennial but will not make it through a winter with below-freezing temperatures.

Lavender doesn't like its roots consistently wet. It prefers and will thrive in well-drained soil in a sunny area. In winter the plant will wither and dry out, actually looking quite dead. Give it time in spring to "wake up" and you will see new little shoots of the plant. Once these shoots start to grow, cut away the old dead stems from last year.

Harvesting

To harvest lavender, cut the stems the clusters of buds are on before they open. Strip the leaves off the stems (these may be dried and used in insect repellent sachets) and tie the lavender stems in a bundle, hanging it upside down to dry. Store whole or strip the buds off the stems.

Growing at a Glance

Optimal Growing Conditions: Well-drained soil, full sun

Will Grow in Zone: 4 to 10; it must be brought in to overwinter in Zone 3. The best lavender choice for Zones 8 to 10 is *L. stoechas.*

Common Propagation: Cuttings for all lavender varieties, seeds for "Lady" and "Munstead" lavender

Type of Plant: Perennial

Used in: Bath Garden (page 88), Children's Herb Garden (page 92), Headache Relief Garden (page 116), Relaxation Garden (page 132), and Skin Care Garden (page 136)

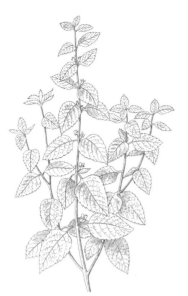

Lemon Balm *(Melissa officinalis)*

Melissa is a Greek word meaning "bee" or "related to the bee." It is an aptly named plant, for the bees love it when it is in bloom. It has been grown for well over two thousand years; the Greeks used lemon balm medicinally by steeping the foliage in wine then drinking it for relief of fevers. The Arabs felt it was good for heart disorders and lifting the spirits. In the 18th century lemon balm was put into elixirs that were supposed to give everlasting youth. It was a common plant in colonial American gardens; Thomas Jefferson grew it in his gardens at Monticello.

Medicinal Uses

This wonderfully lemon-scented plant has sedative, antidepressant, digestive, stimulant, diaphoretic, relaxant, carminative, antiviral, and antispasmodic properties. It should be plain that lemon balm has many uses. Scientific studies have shown that the herb does indeed calm nerves and relieve spasms. It is an uplifting plant used in infusions to promote relaxation, relieve headaches, or help promote sleep. From an aromatic standpoint, the fragrant lemon scent will also help lift the spirits.

An important use of lemon balm is as an antispasmodic to soothe and calm, relieving dyspepsia and nausea, and acting as a digestive aid. I have a friend who has been plagued with gastrointestinal upsets for several years. She has been to doctors, had all of the tests, and taken lots of prescription drugs with little relief. Then I took her some dried lemon balm from my garden, and she started drinking it in an infusion a couple of times a day. She called me to happily report that it does bring her some relief. Now we can't keep her supplied with enough dried lemon balm!

Lemon balm has some topical uses. Crush the fresh leaf and rub it on the skin to relieve insect bites and as an insect repellent. Made into a salve, it can be used on minor scrapes and cuts. Due to its antiviral properties, research and trials are also being done to investigate the use of lemon balm in cream form to treat cold sores and fever blisters.

Lemon balm can also be used to impart a lemon scent and flavor to food. Look for it in herb cookbooks, particularly in baked goods recipes.

As with other herbs, use lemon balm in moderation. There is a small percentage of the population that could suffer from an allergy to lemon balm.

RAISING LEMON BALM

Lemon balm is easily started from seeds. In fact, it readily reseeds itself from the mature plants at the end of its blooming phase, so that you'll find little lemon balm seedlings in all kinds of interesting places in your garden.

The plant likes full sun but will grow in partial shade. It is tolerant of poor weather and soil conditions. The seeds need light to germinate, so, when you're planting, leave them uncovered; just scratch them into the surface of the bed. They can be planted 2 to 3 weeks before the last spring frost, so it is unnecessary to start the seeds any earlier for transplanting into your garden. If you have friends who grows herbs, ask them for a lemon-balm division. I can almost guarantee that they will happily share.

Lemon balm is a member of the mint family, but spreads more slowly than many mints. The 2- to 2½-foot-tall plants will grow into a large clump, with little seedlings sprouting up wherever seeds fall from the small, pretty white-and-green blossoms.

Harvesting

Harvest the leaves and their small tender stems to use. This harvesting will also encourage bushiness and new growth in the plants. After drying, store the leaves in a glass container away from heat and light. The leaves will darken during the drying process. Do not crumble the leaves until you are ready to use them.

Growing at a Glance

Optimal Growing Conditions: Sunny, well-drained soil
Will Grow in Zone: 5 to 10; may be grown as an annual in Zone 4
Common Propagation: Seeds, division
Type of Plant: Perennial
Used in: Bath Garden (page 88), Headache Relief Garden (page 116), Relaxation Garden (page 132), Tummy Care Garden (page 152), and Woman's Care Garden (page 156)

A MULTIPURPOSE INFUSION

A lemon balm infusion is good for headache relief, tension relief, or as an aid to alleviate gastrointestinal distress. To make the infusion, combine 2 teaspoons dried lemon balm leaves, or 4 teaspoons fresh, with 1 cup boiling water. Cover to prevent the essential oils from escaping and let steep for 10 to 15 minutes.

Sip the infusion slowly.

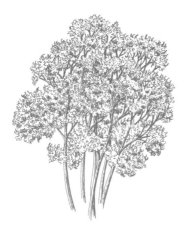

Parsley *(Petroselinum crispum, P. crispum* var. *neapolitanum)*

Parsley is a lovely green plant that has been long admired. The ancient Greeks decorated their tombs and warhorses with it; it also figured heavily into their funeral ceremonies. Romans wore garlands of parsley around their necks at banquets, hoping to have the herb absorb the alcohol fumes and thus stave off drunkenness. They also took parsley with them to Britain, from whence it made its way eventually to North America. Colonial American gardens contained parsley. Unfortunately, parsley has most recently been relegated to nothing more than garnish on a dinner plate.

Medicinal Uses

It is a shame that, by many, parsley is considered only decorative, for this useful plant has stomachic, mild diuretic, mild antiseptic, and carminative properties. Most important, it is extremely nutritious. One cup of chopped parsley contains more beta-carotene than a large carrot, almost twice as much vitamin C as an orange, more calcium than a cup of milk, and 20 times as much iron as one serving of liver. In addition to all of this, it contains phosphorus and potassium. Parsley's high chlorophyll content makes it a perfect after-meal breath freshener. Parsley can also be crushed up and used as a poultice on minor wounds and insect bites.

PARSLEY PESTO

This is an uncommon, yet tasty and very nutritious way to fix parsley. Use as pasta topping or as a spread for Italian bread. It can be prepared ahead and frozen.

1 cup fresh Italian parsley leaves
½ cup fresh caraway thyme
3 garlic cloves, peeled
⅓ cup freshly grated Parmesan cheese
½ cup pine nuts
½ cup extra-virgin olive oil
¾ teaspoon salt (or to taste)
Freshly ground black pepper to taste

Place all ingredients in a food processor and blend until the mixture is well chopped and blended.

Cautions

Don't eat large quantities of parsley if you have kidney problems; it contains an oil that can irritate the kidneys. Don't take large quantities of parsley if you are pregnant; it is an emmenagogue and will stimulate menstruation.

RAISING PARSLEY

Start seeds early for spring parsley plants, because they take a long time to germinate. I usually plant parsley seeds in early spring. To hasten germination, some people soak the seeds in water for 24 hours prior to planting, discarding the water, but I have never found this to be helpful. Just plant the seeds and cover ¼ inch deep with a starting mixture, keep them moist, and be patient. Eventually you will see little grasslike seedlings, which will soon develop the characteristic green foliage.

Transplanting parsley is considered by many to be bad luck, but if you do so, transplant in late spring into deeply worked soil in full to partial sun. Parsley will tolerate mild frost. Grow an extra plant or two for the butterfly caterpillars, because they like to feed on the foliage and will become beautiful butterflies later in the season.

Parsley plants grow to be about 18 to 24 inches high and 10 to 12 inches wide. Curly parsley is very decorative with its rounded bushy form and seems to be preferred by landscapers. Italian parsley is a darker, glossier green with flat leaves and grows a couple of inches taller than the curly-leafed variety. I think Italian parsley has better flavor, but opinions on the subject vary. Taste each variety, and grow whichever you like the best.

In fall, pot up one or two plants to keep you supplied with fresh parsley for winter. Use a deep container to accommodate parsley's deep taproot. Any plants left in the garden will green up come spring and develop their blooms the second year. Leave these in your garden; the umbels will attract beneficial insects and butterflies. I have occasionally had parsley reseed itself at the end of the second year — but don't count on this.

Harvesting

Parsley is best eaten fresh. Dried parsley tastes like it looks — papery. It will put green flecks in your food but is a poor substitute for fresh. Harvest the fresh leaves around the outside of the plant first. If you don't bring any plants in for winter, you can chop and freeze parsley for later use.

Growing at a Glance

Optimal Growing Conditions: Full to partial sun, moist rich soil
Will Grow in Zone: 4 to 8; may be grown as an annual in Zone 3 and Zones 8 to 10
Common Propagation: Seeds
Type of Plant: Biennial
Used in: Mouth Care Garden (page 124) and Rejuvenation Garden (page 128)

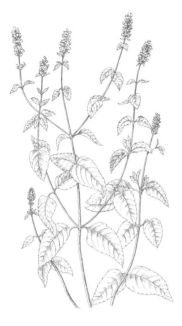

Peppermint *(Mentha x piperita)*

While traveling through northern Indiana on our way home from vacation one year, we drove past fields of plants that didn't look like a typical Indiana farm crop. I asked my husband to pull over so I could take a closer look. When I got out of the car, I was assailed with an aroma that reminded me of candy canes. What we were seeing was fields of peppermint, grown as a cash crop and harvested to obtain the essential oils.

Peppermint appeared as a sterile crossbreed in the late 1600s in England, so any history of the plant starts there. However, the mint cousins — such as spearmint and watermint — from which it derived have been around through the ages. The Egyptian Pharisees paid tithes to the pharaoh with mint; in the early medical record known as Egyptian Ebers Papyrus of 1550 B.C., it was recommended that mint tea be used to alleviate indigestion. In Greece soldiers rubbed their weapons with mint before battle for good luck. The Romans chewed mint after meals, and, as with other herbs that they used, took it with them when they moved, thus spreading mint to other parts of the world.

In early Christian times the herb was such a valuable medicinal that the church accepted it as a payment of tithes. Medieval Europeans used it as a strewing herb and rubbed it on their teeth for fresh breath. They also used the herb to relieve toothaches. Colonists in North America grew mint in their gardens, and there it has grown ever since.

Medicinal Uses

Peppermint's useful properties include carminative, antispasmodic, aromatic, diaphoretic, antiseptic, analgesic, and nervine. Peppermint's volatile oil contains menthol, an ingredient that is familiar to us in many products. It is known to relax visceral muscles. Peppermint contains calcium, vitamins A and C, and riboflavin. The aroma is considered to encourage alertness and wakefulness.

You can use peppermint infusions to relieve a variety of digestive-tract ailments; they stimulate bile production, thereby enhancing digestive activity. They will also help relieve gas and accompanying abdominal pain. The volatile oil acts as a mild anesthetic to the stomach wall, helping decrease nausea and vomiting.

Externally, peppermint stimulates cold-perceiving nerves below the surface of the skin. It can relieve itching and be useful for easing achy muscles. If you're feverish, drinking a peppermint infusion will help you feel better. Peppermint's cooling effects can also be helpful in the summer months when you add the herb to your bathwater.

For an infusion of peppermint, place 1 teaspoon of the dried herb in 1 cup of boiling water and let it steep for 5 to 7 minutes, covered.

Cautions

Be careful, because large amounts of peppermint tea can inhibit the absorption of iron in severely anemic people and can be toxic. Don't give peppermint tea to babies and small children — the volatile oils can cause them to have a choking sensation.

RAISING PEPPERMINT

Just saying the above two words — raising peppermint — is a gross understatement given peppermint's propensity to grow. Like its other mint relatives, once peppermint is planted in a favorable area, it will grow and spread to an amazing degree. The first year I planted mine, it went from one tiny stem to a 1½-foot clump. The next year it grew to a patch about 4 feet around.

Beware of any packages of seeds that claim to be peppermint; this plant is sterile, so you must start it from cuttings or division. It's best to pick a spot where peppermint can spread out. To contain it, plant in a large (12-inch-diameter or larger) container and sink into the ground, if desired. I let all of my mints grow as they will, taking a shovel or garden fork and digging out clumps around the edges to contain them. These clumps easily can be divided and potted up for plant or garage sales or for hands-on lessons for gardening students learning to divide plants.

Peppermint will grow in very moist conditions without complaint. Its light requirements are sun to partial shade. The plant has attractive purplish stems that grow to be 18 inches to 2½ feet tall. Its lavender blooms appear in late summer.

Harvesting

To harvest peppermint, cut the stems and dry the leaves while still attached. Ideally you'll do this before the plants bloom. When they are dry, use your fingers to strip the leaves from the stems, and store in a glass container away from heat and light.

Growing at a Glance

Optimal Growing Conditions: Moist rich soil, sun to partial shade

Will Grow in Zone: 4 to 10; may be grown as an annual in Zone 3, or brought in as a container plant

Common Propagation: Division, cuttings

Type of Plant: Perennial

Used in: Bath Garden (page 88), Cold and Flu Garden (page 96), and Tummy Care Garden (page 152)

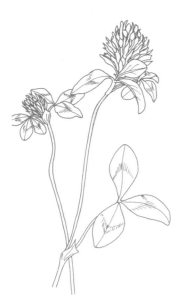

Red Clover *(Trifolium pratense)*

From my childhood on a farm in central Indiana, I have a clear memory of red clover. It grew in many fields where the livestock grazed. It was also cut and harvested for hay, an aroma that I still find extremely pleasant and associate with hot summer days. I also remember the aroma of the clusters of pink-rose blooms, and how sweet the ends of each tiny pink flower tasted when I chewed them. Back then, I never would have given a thought to using the flowers for anything else.

Red clover was revered by the ancient Greeks, Romans, and Celts. Early Christians linked the plant to the holy trinity due to the configuration of its leaves. When the plant was introduced to America, the Natives used it medicinally.

Medicinal Uses

I am not sure exactly when red clover was recognized as a useful medicinal plant. Probably — as is so often the case — people discovered by trial and error that this beautiful plant can help treat many ailments. Its properties are relaxant, expectorant, antispasmodic, and diuretic; it acts as an internal cleanser. It has been claimed to be an appetite suppressant, but I believe that if red clover truly worked in this way it would have swept the country as a natural diet aid by now. The herb also contains vitamins A, B, and C, and the minerals calcium and phosphorus.

A pleasant infusion made from the blossoms may relieve coughs due to colds and promote relaxation for people suffering from colds and flu. An infusion can be given safely to children: Use 1 teaspoon of the dried blossoms to 1 cup of boiling water, covering while it steeps for 10 to 15 minutes. Adults can use 2 to 3 teaspoons of the dried blossoms to 1 cup of boiling water. It makes a delicate and slightly fragrant infusion that is pleasant to sip on. Only drink 1 to 3 cups of the infusion per day.

Its cleansing and diuretic properties have made red clover a popular treatment to assist in clearing up skin disorders and eczema. Give a cup of the infusion to a teen in your family who is concerned about his or her complexion.

Red clover is in the legume family. Legumes contain compounds called isoflavones that aid in regulating the immune system. Research done by the National Cancer Institute has found possible antitumor properties in red clover.

Cautions

An autumn harvest of red clover has resulted in gastrointestinal disturbances in animals, so harvest it in the summertime for human consumption. Do not use if you are pregnant or taking blood-thinning medications.

RAISING RED CLOVER

Red clover is started easily from seeds. The little plants quickly will grow into bushy clumps about 1½ feet in diameter and 2 feet high. The blooms will appear the next season, although I have seen some plants bloom the first season. If you leave the blooms on the plants to dry, red clover will reseed itself, giving you a continuous crop of red clover. If you cut back the plants near the end of their first blooming, they will bloom again for a later-summer harvest. Don't forget to use the cuttings for a most useful addition to your compost pile.

As a legume, red clover will fix nitrogen by obtaining nitrogen from the air and transferring it to the soil, enhancing the soil quality. It is also a good green-manure crop sown in fall or early spring, then tilled into the soil before it blooms. (Green manure is plant material grown to dig back into the soil to improve fertility and add to the organic content.)

Harvesting

Harvest clover just as the blooms are fully open. Check the plants daily for new blooms. Harvesting them can be time consuming, because the blooms continue coming on for several weeks. You must be diligent in gathering them. Dry the blooms with gentle heat and store in a glass container away from heat and light.

Growing at a Glance

Optimal Growing Conditions: Full sun, rich soil
Will Grow in Zone: 5 to 9
Common Propagation: Seeds
Type of Plant: Biennial
Used in: Rejuvenation Garden (page 128) and Woman's Care Garden (page 156)

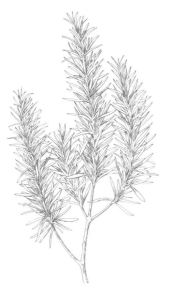

Rosemary *(Rosmarinus officinalis)*

This is probably my favorite herb for cooking and using medicinally. I grow so much of it that, in the cold months, my windowsills are full of rosemary plants.

Greek students wore rosemary in garlands on their heads when they were taking exams; they felt that it improved their memory. Medieval households used rosemary-scented water for hand washing. It was believed that rosemary refused to grow in gardens of evil people, an idea that is disconcerting to me given that there have been some years when I can't keep a single plant alive! In the Middle Ages people carried sprigs of rosemary in their pockets to ward off evil spirits, and placed sprigs under their pillows at night to prevent nightmares.

Rosemary has been burned in sick chambers to purify the air, and branches were strewn in law courts to protect those present from jail fever, also known as typhus. Likewise, during the Middle Ages it was believed that the reason rosemary's flowers are blue is because the Virgin Mary had laid her blue cloak across the rosemary bush when it was in bloom, coloring the flowers. The herb was woven into bridal wreaths as a symbol of fidelity and constancy. Rosemary's natural antioxidant properties slow food spoilage and made it appropriate for food preservation in the days before refrigeration.

Medicinal Uses

Rosemary contains antioxidant, antiviral, carminative, antibacterial, anti-inflammatory, and circulatory stimulant properties. Recent research has shown that rosemary enhances the cell's intake of oxygen, which would aid in cerebral function. Rosemary contains calcium, magnesium, phosphorus, sodium, potassium, and vitamins A and C.

Make rosemary-infused oil (see page 12) to use as a sore muscle rub. The infused oil will stimulate blood circulation to affected areas. Or make a rosemary infusion of 1 cup dried rosemary to 2 quarts boiling water for external use. Cover and steep for 10 minutes, then strain. Add the 2 quarts of infusion to a basin of water, adjusting the temperature to warm. Use as a soak to relieve tired, achy feet. Add this strained infusion to your bath for a stimulating soak.

For a housewide inhalant, simmer the above infusion in a pan on the stove, allowing the aroma of rosemary to travel throughout your home, helping clear the cold-related nasal and chest congestion of everyone within. For external use, make an infusion of 2 tablespoons dried rosemary or 4 tablespoons fresh to 1 cup boiling water. Cover and let steep for 10 minutes, then strain. Cool to room temperature and use as a facial rinse after cleansing or a hair rinse after shampooing.

For an infusion to be taken internally, use 1 teaspoon of dried herb to 1 cup of water. Let steep for 10 minutes, then strain and sip slowly.

Cautions

Due to its stimulating properties, rosemary should only be used as an internal infusion at a maximum of 2 cups a day for no longer than a week at a time. People with high blood pressure should avoid use of rosemary in other than a culinary way.

RAISING ROSEMARY

There are several ways to grow rosemary. One is by taking cuttings; another is to layer a low-lying stem into the soil where the plant is growing. These two methods are best for any variety of rosemary, but a third way is by starting plants from seeds. Common rosemary or *Rosmarinus officinalis* can be started from seeds with a little care. After barely covering the seeds with starting mix, mist the soil daily to prevent a crust from forming over them. Plant more seeds than you will want plants, for the germination rate is low. After the seedlings have emerged, continue misting them.

Rosemary is tender and will not survive outdoors in areas that receive frost. To keep it alive, take cuttings of plants to raise indoors, or dig up plants from the ground and move to pots when temperatures turn cool.

Allow container-grown rosemary to dry out between waterings. The plants will enjoy a daily misting, particularly in homes with low humidity. A lot of people think their rosemary is dead when the leaves resemble those of a parched Christmas tree. My answer is to water the plant and wait a day to see what happens. Chances are good that it will perk up.

Harvesting

To harvest rosemary, cut off the stems of the plant and allow the leaves to become crumbly dry. Strip the leaves from the stems, and place them in a glass container away from light or heat for storage.

Growing at a Glance

Optimal Growing Conditions: Medium to rich well-drained soil, warm temperatures

Will Grow in Zone: 8 to 10; in other zones you must treat rosemary as an annual or place in containers for wintering indoors

Common Propagation: Cuttings

Type of Plant: Tender perennial

Used in: Bath Garden (page 88), Cold and Flu Garden (page 96), Decongestant Garden (page 100), Hair Care Garden (page 112), Skin Care Garden (page 136), Sore Muscle Care Garden (page 140), and Windowsill Medicine Cabinet (page 160)

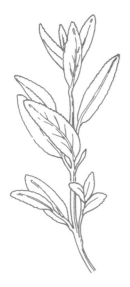

Sage *(Salvia officinalis)*

The word *salvia* means "to save," and throughout history many people believed that sage saved them from various ills. Arabian people felt that sage increased longevity — an old Arab proverb asks, "How can a man die who has sage in his garden?" It is thought that King Solomon's gardens grew sage. Medieval monastery gardens included sage. The Chinese were so impressed with this herb that they were willing to trade three chests of their tea for one chest of sage. It was grown in colonial gardens and used prolifically to help preserve food due to its antibacterial properties. To some, sage symbolizes immortality, wisdom, and longevity.

Medicinal Uses

The usefulness of sage is not just imagined. Sage has carminative, spasmolytic, antiseptic, astringent, antibiotic, antibacterial, stimulant, tonic, and antihidrotic properties. The herb contains vitamins A, B, and C, niacin, potassium, calcium, and iron.

Sage's astringent and antiseptic properties will help relieve a sore throat and mouth. Along with professional medical care, a gargle of sage infusion will assist in healing any inflammation that is present.

When taken internally, sage decreases the amount of perspiration your body excretes. It will also decrease salivation and lactation. Sage stimulates the gastrointestinal tract, relieves indigestion, and aids in the digestion of fatty foods. This truly makes it a good addition to large meals, and is probably why sage has traditionally been included in recipes for holiday feasts.

For a home air purifier, place a bit of dried sage on a heatproof surface and light it. The smoke from the burning sage will cleanse the air. Some varieties of sage and artemisias are used to make smudge sticks, which are used in Native American rituals in an act of purification.

Cautions

Sage can stimulate the central nervous system and contains thujone, a dangerous toxic substance that can trigger seizures. Anyone with a seizure disorder should avoid using sage in anything but small culinary amounts. You should also avoid taking sage when pregnant except, again, in small culinary amounts. Sage also interferes with the absorption of iron. If you are taking an iron preparation and/or are suffering from some form of anemia, avoid taking sage. Do not ingest sage in large amounts or over a prolonged period of time.

RAISING SAGE

Common sage *(Salvia officinalis)* is easy to start from seeds. Start them indoors in well-drained starting mix; fresh seeds germinate more easily than older. I start my seed in early to midspring. When the seedlings emerge, usually in 2 to 3 weeks, they will have the characteristically wrinkled leaves of the adult plants. You can set the new plants out early, because they will tolerate a frost. Sage likes full sun and well-drained soil, but it will tolerate poor soils. It is remarkably drought resistant and will still be holding up well when other plants in your garden are looking droopy during dry weather. A sage plant will grow into a large 12-inch-tall clump that will become full sized in 2 years. It will have spikes of purplish blue blooms early in summer. The leaves stay green and usable most of early winter, so you can use fresh sage in holiday recipes.

Sage can also be started by cuttings and layering. There are several kinds of sage with foliage of different sizes and colors. I have found in my gardens that the most colorful sages — purple sage, golden sage, or tricolored sage — will not survive winter. Propagate these varieties by cuttings or layering, and grow in a sheltered place for overwintering.

When cared for properly, a sage plant will live quite a few years. I had one that grew for 8 or 9 years before it became woody and the amount of foliage decreased. Sage can get leggy and unattractive in containers indoors for winter. I usually harvest fresh leaves until the severe cold of midwinter causes the plant to die back; then I use my dried supply.

Harvesting

To harvest sage, cut stems full of leaves above leaf joint or node. Allow to dry. When the leaves are crumbly, store in a glass container away from heat and light. Do not crumble up the leaves until you are ready to use them.

Growing at a Glance

Optimal Growing Conditions:
Full sun, well-drained soil
Will Grow in Zone:
4 to 7; will not overwinter in Zone 3, and develops rot in Zones 8 to 10 — plant in raised beds
Common Propagation:
Seeds, cuttings
Type of Plant: Perennial
Used in: Hair Care Garden (page 112), Mouth Care Garden (page 124), and Throat Care Garden (page 144)

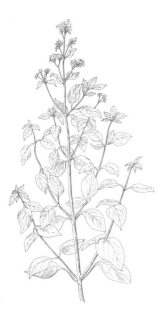

Sweet Marjoram *(Origanum majorana)*

This intensely spicy-scented herb was supposedly created by the Greek goddess Aphrodite as a symbol of happiness. Oil infused with marjoram was massaged into the foreheads and hair of ancient Greeks after their baths, possibly to improve blood flow to those areas. They also believed that if marjoram grew on a tomb, the deceased person was happy. The plant was introduced to Europe in the Middle Ages. A book written in the late 14th century by an older wealthy Parisian to his young wife included a description of how to use marjoram in washing water. It was used as a fragrant strewing herb. The fragrant oil has been used as an ingredient in soaps and perfumes for many years.

Medicinal Uses

Marjoram has antioxidant, carminative, diaphoretic, antispasmodic, sedative, antiseptic, and tonic properties. It also contains vitamins A and C, calcium, phosphorus, iron, and magnesium.

Sip an infusion of 1 teaspoon dried herb or 2 teaspoons fresh to 1 cup of boiling water, covered and steeped for 10 minutes, to relieve symptoms of a cold. The same cup of infusion can be soothing to jangled nerves and help relieve stress and tension. The carminative and antispasmodic properties of a marjoram infusion will aid in relieving simple gastrointestinal upsets. Singers are known to drink a marjoram infusion with honey in it to prevent hoarseness. The infusion can also be used as an antiseptic lotion for troubled skin.

Do use caution in trying marjoram preparations, since a small percentage of the population might be allergic to this herb.

SORE MUSCLE REMEDY

An infused oil of marjoram (see page 12) makes a great massage oil for sprains and sore muscles. A strong infusion of marjoram added to a bathtub of warm water makes a beneficial soak for tired and sore muscles. To prepare a strong infusion, steep ½ cup of dried herb, or 1 cup fresh, in 2 quarts of boiling water for 10 minutes. Strain out the herbs and let the liquid cool to lukewarm, then add it to your warm bathwater.

RAISING SWEET MARJORAM

Starting marjoram from seeds is very easy: 6 to 10 weeks before your last frost date, plant the seeds indoors in moist starting mix and barely cover them. In a few days you will have little marjoram seedlings that will rapidly grow. Transplant the new plants outside after all danger of frost is over. Marjoram does best in full sun with moderately rich soil, although it will grow in heavier soils without much difficulty. The plants are tolerant of slightly alkaline soil.

Mature plants will be about 8 to 10 inches tall and slightly sprawling to about 6 inches in diameter. The blooms look like little green knots on the stems, giving the plant an interesting look that will add contrast to your garden. If you do not live in a frost-free climate, treat marjoram as an annual. Or, you can grow marjoram in containers for winter use. It will sprawl a bit, causing it to spill over the side of its container.

Harvesting

Harvest marjoram by cutting stems, with the leaves still attached, about halfway down. Dry, then strip the leaves from the stems. Store in a tightly closed glass container away from heat and light.

Growing at a Glance

Optimal Growing Conditions: Full sun, well-drained soil

Will Grow in Zone: 9 to 10 as a perennial; treat as an annual in all other growing zones

Common Propagation: Seeds

Type of Plant: Tender perennial

Used in: Bath Garden (page 88), Relaxation Garden (page 132), Sore Muscle Care Garden (page 140), Throat Care Garden (page 144), Tummy Care Garden (page 152), and Windowsill Medicine Cabinet (page 160)

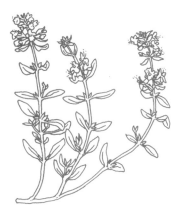

Thyme *(Thymus vulgaris)*

I didn't have thyme in my gardens the first couple of years that I grew herbs; I wasn't convinced that this little shrubby plant was worth growing. If I had read up on its history, though, I would've realized what a useful plant it was and still is.

The ancient Greek physician Hippocrates and his contemporaries prized thyme highly for its medicinal qualities. In Greece a supreme compliment was to say that someone "smelled of thyme." It was burned as incense in ancient Greek temples. In ancient Rome thyme was burned as deodorizer, and Roman soldiers bathed in it for vigor. The Egyptians used it medicinally, too. The crusaders brought the seeds home with them, and thyme became a common addition to their families' gardens and households. The herb was used for strewing, and an infusion was used to combat excessive body lice.

Thyme's essential oil is strongly antiseptic, and during World War I it was used for that reason. During various times in history thyme has been used for such diverse complaints as colic, melancholia, sore throat, insomnia, nightmares, hangovers, and alcohol addiction. Thyme symbolizes health, healing, sleep, psychic powers, love, purification, and courage.

Medicinal Uses

Thyme's properties are carminative, antimicrobial, antispasmodic, expectorant, stimulant, relaxant, and astringent. Research done in Japan shows thyme works as an antioxidant as well. It contains vitamins A and D, niacin, phosphorus, potassium, calcium, iron, magnesium, and zinc.

Thyme's best medicinal use, in my opinion, is as an adjunct in treating sore throats, colds, and congestion. An infusion made from the herb will help soothe a sore throat and act as an expectorant, due to an active constituent found in thyme called thymol. German studies have found thyme to be effective for the treatment of symptoms of bronchitis, coughs, and colds. To make an infusion, add 1 teaspoon dried thyme or 2 teaspoons fresh to 1 cup boiling water. Cover and steep the infusion for 10 minutes, then strain. Adding honey increases the infusion's effectiveness.

Thyme's antimicrobial property makes it a good choice for use in skin care. An infusion of the leaves and flowers can be used as a facial lotion for blemished skin. To make a lotion, put 2 tablespoons dried herb or 4 tablespoons fresh in 1 cup of boiling water, then cover and steep for 10 minutes. Cool before using. Including thyme in herbal bath mixtures can add a deodorizing quality to your bath, as well as releasing the aroma for an inhalation to relieve colds and congestion.

Cautions

Do not ingest thyme other than in culinary amounts if you have thyroid problems. If you have high blood pressure, avoid using thyme except for culinary use. Avoid using large amounts of thyme if you are pregnant. Do not give thyme preparations to children under the age of 3 years.

RAISING THYME

There is a multitude of thyme varieties of different aromas, heights, and foliage colors, which makes thyme a good plant to include in garden planning. For optimal use of thyme's healing properties, however, common thyme or *Thymus vulgaris* is the best choice. Thyme is low growing and makes a nice border for a garden. People used to plant it for the fairies to live under, and no wonder: It is just the right size for them!

Starting common thyme from seeds is trouble-free. Plant the seeds indoors in early spring, barely covering them, and give them an environment of around 70°F (21°C) in which to germinate. Mist the top of the soil to keep it moist and prevent crusting over. Transplant the seedlings when the weather is warm and the danger of heavy frost is past. Give thyme a sunny spot with well-drained soil in which to grow and you will be rewarded with 8- to 12-inch-tall plants that will expand to about 12 inches high, looking like little shrubs. The tiny, prolific pale lavender flowers are quite beautiful and will attract bees to your garden to help pollinate your plants. Thyme will stay green in all but the coldest months of winter, and it will never need watering, not even in the driest months of summer.

This herb can also be propagated by cuttings and layering. Often the lowermost branches will touch the ground and layer themselves, giving you starts for additional plants. This season I even had some thyme self-seed; I found new little seedlings sprouting in the cracks of the stepping-stones in my garden. Thyme can be grown in containers and brought in for winter availability of the fresh herb. It does tend to get leggy when grown indoors.

Harvesting

Thyme's active properties are at their peak just as the plant is coming into bloom. To harvest, cut the stems about halfway down and dry them. Strip the leaves and flowers and store in a tightly covered glass container away from heat and light.

Growing at a Glance

Optimal Growing Conditions: Full sun, well-drained soil
Will Grow in Zone: 4 to 7; treat as an annual in Zones 3 and 8 to 10
Common Propagation: Seeds, layering, cuttings
Type of Plant: Perennial
Used in: Bath Garden (page 88), Children's Herb Garden (page 92), Cold and Flu Garden (page 96), Mouth Care Garden (page 124), Throat Care Garden (page 144), and Windowsill Medicine Cabinet (page 160)

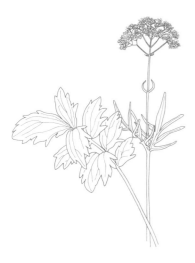

Valerian *(Valeriana officinalis)*

Remember the story of the Pied Piper of Hamelin? It is rumored that besides his music, he used valerian to help lure the rats out of the town.

The word *valerian* comes from the Latin word *valere,* which means "to be in health." Used as early as the 4th century B.C. by Hippocrates, valerian was found to help calm tension and stress. It was considered valuable enough to be brought to the New World by European colonists. Valerian symbolizes love, sleep, purification, and protection.

During World Wars I and II, valerian was given to soldiers suffering from shell shock and nervous stress. Although widely used in this country in the first half of the 20th century, valerian-based medicines are no longer available here. The herb is, however, the most widely used sedative in Germany.

Medicinal Uses

Valerian has sedative, hypnotic, antispasmodic, hypotensive, and carminative properties. Studies have shown that it acts as a relaxant on the central nervous system. This makes it helpful for use in reducing tension and anxiety, and calming excitability. Its relaxing effect can also be helpful in promoting sleep. It has been found to have a greater sedative effect than lemon balm. (See page 42.) Use the roots to obtain the active constituents. Do not confuse *Valeriana officinalis* with red valerian, a common perennial that has no medicinal value.

Dried or steeped valerian roots have an odor that most people find unpleasant. An infusion made from the roots not only smells bad, but is also bitter. In addition, some of the active ingredients are not water soluble. To use, make your own capsules by chopping up the dried roots and placing them in size 00 gelatin capsules (available at natural-food stores). Take two capsules at night to promote sleep.

Cautions

Taking two valerian capsules daily for longer than 2 to 3 weeks can lead to headaches and heart palpitations. Valerian enhances the action of sleep-inducing drugs; don't take the two substances at the same time. Be aware that some people respond to valerian as a stimulant. Alcohol and valerian don't mix; the two combined can lead to potentially dangerous depression of the central nervous system.

TINCTURE OF VALERIAN

Make a tincture using a ratio of 2 tablespoons dried valerian root to 2 cups of pure grain alcohol or good-quality vodka and 2 cups distilled water (see page 13). The recommended dosage for promoting sleep is 10 to 20 drops of the tincture at night. Do not use the tincture for more than a 2- to 3-week period.

RAISING VALERIAN

Valerian can be started easily from seeds, as evidenced by little plants you'll see around the adults when you leave the flowers to go to seed. Stratify the seeds for 3 weeks prior to planting. (See page 165.) I start the seeds indoors. They need light to germinate, so don't cover them; just place them on top of your starting mix. Plant them outside as soon as the danger of heavy frost is past.

The adult plants slowly spread and can be divided every 3 years. Valerian appreciates rich, moist soil and full sun, but it will grow in lesser soils and partial shade. If you have cats, they will hover around when you are dividing and planting valerian, because they like the smell of the roots.

Keep in mind that the adult plants are 4 to 5 feet tall, so place them in the back of border plantings. Richly scented clusters of white flowers will bloom once warm weather arrives.

Harvesting

To harvest, dig the roots in late fall, leaving enough plants to reproduce and give you subsequent crops. Clean the roots thoroughly and dry them slowly. Once they're dry, store in a glass container away from heat and light.

Growing at a Glance

Optimal Growing Conditions: Full sun, rich well-worked soil
Will Grow in Zone: 4 to 8
Common Propagation: Seeds, division
Type of Plant: Perennial
Used in: Relaxation Garden (page 132)

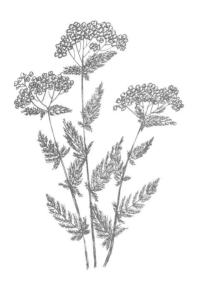

Yarrow *(Achillea millefolium)*

Yarrow is said to be named for the ancient hero Achilles, who was supposed to have used the herb to treat his wounded soldiers. Yarrow was indeed a popular wound treatment for the ancient Greeks, and continued to be popular into the mid-19th century, when it was used by field doctors in the American Civil War to treat wounds. The Chinese used the stalks of the yarrow plant to make I Ching predictions, a method of answering questions about the future. Native Americans used yarrow to halt bleeding and promote wound healing. It's not known whether European settlers introduced yarrow to the New World or the Natives used a plant already here. Nevertheless, it is quite a useful plant. It symbolizes courage, love, and psychic powers to some.

Medicinal Uses

Yarrow's properties are diaphoretic, hypotensive, astringent, antiseptic, hemostatic, and anti-inflammatory. Historically, one of yarrow's most popular uses was as a wound treatment. To treat a minor cut or scrape that is bleeding, take a clean leaf or two of yarrow, crush it, and apply to the wound. The hemostatic and antiseptic properties should help to stop the bleeding and promote healing.

Its diaphoretic property gives yarrow the reputation of being helpful in feverish conditions. Make an infusion of 1 to 2 teaspoons of yarrow (you may also mix in equal parts red clover and catnip) and 1 cup of boiling water; cover and infuse for 10 minutes. Sip slowly. Drink no more than 3 cups of the infusion a day.

YARROW SKIN TONER

Yarrow's astringent and antiseptic properties make it useful as a toner for those suffering from oily skin. Make an infusion of 1 to 2 teaspoons steeped for 10 minutes in 1 cup boiling water. Apply the infusion to the skin after cleansing. You can keep this skin toner in the refrigerator for 48 hours. Don't forget to try the patch test (see page 10) before using it.

Cautions

Taking too much yarrow over a prolonged period of time can cause headaches and vertigo. As with all herbs, moderation is in order. Yarrow ingestion can interfere with the absorption of iron and other minerals. When used with other herbs, yarrow can intensify their medicinal actions; consult a qualified herbal practitioner before you do so. Prolonged use of yarrow can make the skin light-sensitive. Since it is a member of the daisy family, do not use it if you have related allergies. Do not ingest yarrow if you are pregnant.

RAISING YARROW

Look around your property and you may not need to raise yarrow. Regarded as a weed by many people, it may be on your land somewhere; move it to a place where you would like to have it growing.

If you don't already have yarrow, it is easy to start. It is very hardy and likes full sun. It will grow in poor soils as well as rich, and is very drought tolerant. Plant the seeds in a spot with full sun after the soil has warmed. Cover them lightly with a little soil. Soon you will see little plants with the characteristic feathery leaves of the adult. Yarrow can also be grown from mature plant divisions.

The beautiful white flowers grow in flat clusters on the plants, attracting butterflies and beneficial insects to your garden. Mature yarrow plants send out runners that will cause the plant to spread. If you don't remove the spent blooms, yarrow will also reseed itself.

Harvesting

Early in the season when yarrow is in full bloom, cut the stems halfway down (above the leaf joint) after the plant has started to bloom. Dry the leaves and flowers on the stems, then strip them off, discarding the stems. Store the dried leaves and flowers in a glass container away from heat and light. Later in the season during the last blooms, cut the stems all the way down to the ground.

Growing at a Glance

Optimal Growing Conditions: Full sun, poor to moderate soil
Will Grow in Zone: 3 to 9
Common Propagation: Seeds, division
Type of Plant: Perennial
Used in: Cold and Flu Garden (page 96), Decongestant Garden (page 100), First Aid Garden (page 108), and Hair Care Garden (page 112)

USDA GROWING ZONE MAP

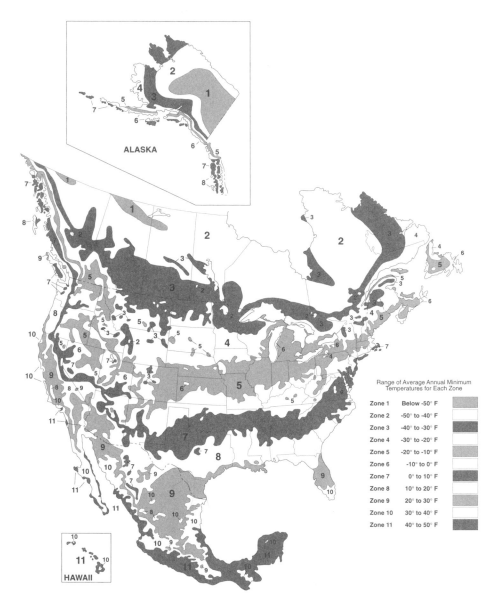

Range of Average Annual Minimum
Temperatures for Each Zone

Zone 1	Below -50° F
Zone 2	-50° to -40° F
Zone 3	-40° to -30° F
Zone 4	-30° to -20° F
Zone 5	-20° to -10° F
Zone 6	-10° to 0° F
Zone 7	0° to 10° F
Zone 8	10° to 20° F
Zone 9	20° to 30° F
Zone 10	30° to 40° F
Zone 11	40° to 50° F

ALASKA

HAWAII

CHAPTER 4

Planning Your Medicinal Herb Garden

Herbal Haiku

Sunshower fondling
Herbal seedlings skyward bound —
Seasonings of life

—*Carol Chau*

When you plant an herb garden you are echoing the actions of gardeners from thousands of years before you. Pliny the Elder of ancient Rome considered herbs important enough to state in his writings that one-quarter of a garden should be set aside for herb growing. Several centuries later, monasteries throughout Europe were primary places for herb gardens. For a number of years, the monks had been keeping herbal knowledge alive by copying herbal manuscripts and employing herbs in a wide array of medicinal uses. The general population would seek out the monks for treatment of their ills. Garlic and thyme were used as antiseptics. Diarrhea was treated with yarrow, plantain, or thyme. Each illness was treated with one or more herbs.

Hortus was the word used to refer to cultivated plots of land that contained a substantial number of herbs. Today the word represents topics related to plants and their growth. In fact, *Hortus* is the title of a thorough reference manual on plants.

Domestic herb gardens were popular in Renaissance Europe. By the early 1500s, instructors who trained doctors felt that medicinal herbs should be available to students for the direct study of the plants. From this idea the first "physic" garden was founded for the study of medicinal plants at a medical school in Padua, Italy.

Herbs are now experiencing a modern-day renaissance. Many of us are not only using herbs, but also rediscovering the multiple pleasures that go along with herb gardening. This chapter will give you some basic gardening information and ideas to help you get started.

PLANNING YOUR GARDEN SITE

Planning ahead will help make your gardening efforts successful. There are many considerations when planning an herb bed. The first one is, of course, availability of space. Whether you live in an apartment or on acres of land, you have to decide where you would like to plant your herbs, along with how many and which kinds to plant. If you have the time, check out potential garden spaces at different times of the day and year. This will give you a lot of information about each site and help you with your choice.

Think seriously about how much time you have to spend gardening, including time for planting and maintenance, before making plans. If you have limited time, then perhaps you should plan a small garden initially. You can work up to more space as your time and interest permit.

Another consideration is how much physical energy you have to garden. This assessment is particularly important if you are older, have physical disabilities, or have a chronic illness. If your energy levels are limited, then perhaps smaller garden spaces or containers would be more manageable.

Educate Yourself

Gardening has become a popular pastime in this country, so there is a lot of information available from a variety of sources. Some resources, including Master Gardeners and local plant nurseries, can offer information on local growing requirements and gardeners. Local libraries usually have a wide variety of gardening and herb-gardening books. Many libraries offer garden-related programs throughout the year. Let your local library know if you are interested in a gardening program.

If you are new to your area or are a brand-new gardener, several resources can give you gardening information. A good place to start is your local County Extension Service office. There you can get information on typical growing conditions for your area, including soil conditions, typical weather patterns, your growing zone, and literature on any number of gardening topics.

Many states' extension services have Master Gardener programs. These classes give valuable gardening information to anyone interested, usually for a small fee; I highly recommend them.

Joining a garden club can put you in touch with people who have similar gardening interests, and give you a group of people with whom to share information. Check your local newspapers for meeting dates and times of garden clubs or similar groups.

Gardening Wisdom
From Leicester, NC

Kate Jayne and her husband, Fairman, own Sandy Mush Herb Nursery, a mail-order plant business. They started growing plants for sale in 1975, and now offer over 1,500 different varieties of herbs and fragrant plants. They have plants suitable for a variety of growing conditions anywhere in the country.

Their soil tends to be porous, acidic loam, but soil tests help them determine how to treat it. "They love it here!" says Kate of their herb plants. She advises that if your soil produces healthy native plants, then herbs such as calendula, catnip, purple coneflower, cayenne pepper, feverfew, red clover, and lavender will do well. She also raises yarrow, parsley, thyme, sage, peppermint, garlic, dill, and fennel with good results.

Kate's special garden tip: "Remember late-spring freezes and the damage they do if the gardener rushes the spring season." (See Resources for more information.)

Learning to Grow

Garden books and magazines are full of pictures of lush, beautiful gardens. Don't be intimidated into thinking that your garden must look exactly like these! It takes some time to get a garden to look picture perfect. Most of us had to start from scratch and learn from our mistakes as we went. If you enjoy growing and using your herbs, that is what counts.

A garden is a flexible thing; it can change with each season, according to your desires. As you read, garden, and learn, you will find plants that you want to try and garden plans that you think are appropriate for your situation. A visit to someone else's garden or a nursery can trigger new ideas. Keep alert to these inspirations. They can lead you into aspects of gardening you hadn't thought about before.

Bigger Is Not Necessarily Better

Start with a small plot of land for herb growing, especially if you are a beginner. The frustrations of overextending yourself in gardening are just as great as in other aspects of life, so begin with just a few herb plants in which you have an interest. This will prove much more satisfying and give you a manageable amount of space to care for. You'll have plenty of time to expand your herbs each gardening season. I have been herb gardening for over a decade and started with a 2-foot by 3-foot raised bed. Every year I expanded my growing space; now I have around 50 herb plants in different places and situations on our property.

LOCATION, LOCATION, LOCATION

Picking a spot for your herb bed involves several criteria. Take a good look around your property, and pick out two or three spots where you might want to plant some herbs. Then monitor the sites for sunlight, drainage, and the shape of the land.

Another important consideration is how close the herb bed is to your house. Try to put it in a place that is easily accessible for care and harvest. You will be much more likely to use your herbs if they are planted where you can quickly run out and harvest some as you need them.

Sunlight

When you're considering a planting spot, look at the amount of sun it receives throughout the day. Sun is a big requirement for a lot of herbs; they need it to produce their essential oils. Most herbs need at least a half day of sunlight. Morning is the best time for the plants to receive sunshine, since this will dry the dew on the leaves and stems, which will help prevent fungal diseases. If you are container-gardening, keep in mind that containers can be placed on roller platforms and moved with the sunlight as needed.

Areas next to your house that receive sun from the southwest can become very hot in the summer. Even heat lovers such as yarrow, echinacea, rosemary, and thyme will wilt when exposed to the unrelenting heat of midday in this position. In this case, a background planting of an ornamental shrub can provide some protection from the midday heat.

Shade

All green plants need some sun for chlorophyll production. A completely shaded spot will probably not support any of the herbs I have discussed. If your land is shaded, look for spots that receive sunlight during some part of the day, or else have dappled shade (dots of sunlight and shade). Many plants appreciate this kind of light because it is not as hot in the sunny afternoons of summer.

If you are not sure whether a spot offers enough sunlight, try placing a few containers of herbs there. If they start to look "leggy" — with long stems and small leaves that seem to be reaching out for sunlight — then most likely the spot doesn't have enough light for your plants to thrive.

Slopes, Terraces, and Wet Land

Slopes can make attractive places for plantings, but cultivating slopes can lead to soil erosion. There are several ways to prevent this. Growing a cover crop between herb plantings can help to prevent erosion. The cover crop, which is a planting of a low-growing variety of plant such as clover, covers the bare ground between established plants. The roots of established plants will help hold soil in place. Mulch heavily around any slope plantings and consider building terraces — steps of soil formed at a perpendicular angle to a sloping piece of land and held in place with supports of wood or stone.

Low places can accumulate water, leading to rotting plants and diseases encouraged by wet conditions. Adding organic matter in large amounts can promote drainage. Chronically wet spots can be turned into planting areas by making raised beds.

Watering

Think about how you want to water the herbs, and whether your planned bed is close enough to a water source for easy maintenance. If your herb bed is

Gardening Wisdom
From Fairbanks, AK

The words Zone 3 and growing sound like a contradiction of terms to me. But, according to Barbara Fay, who teaches classes in growing herbs at the University of Alaska and Georgeson Botanical Gardens in Fairbanks, Alaska, growing herbs is definitely possible. Due to the long, cold winters (temperatures reach −50° to −60°F, or −46° to −51°C), many perennial plants will not survive outdoors and must be brought in or treated as annuals. Another challenge is that the planting season in May and June is dry.

Yarrow and silver thyme will overwinter outdoors for her, but common thyme (*Thymus vulgaris*) does not. Barbara treats parsley as an annual, and digs up sage, sweet marjoram, and lavender to take inside for the winter. She keeps her rosemary in pots year-round for easy relocation indoors. Barbara also direct-seeds dill and fennel and starts lemon balm from seeds, although it will occasionally overwinter for her.

several yards from a water source and you must carry water in a bucket, you will be less likely to water the plants when it is very dry.

There are many different methods of watering plants. Your choices will depend on your garden, your climate, and your budget, among other things. Container gardens in all climates are well suited to the use of a watering can or spray nozzle attachment on a hose. Garden sprinklers can save you time if you have a large garden, and they come in a wide range of prices. Soaker hoses or drip irrigation systems are well-suited to dry climates since they deliver water deeply and directly to the plants' root systems with minimal evaporation.

EVALUATING YOUR CLIMATE

Consider your climate and growing zone as you contemplate locations for your herb bed. If you have cold, windy winters, a sheltered area would be a good choice. If summers are very hot, a spot shaded in the afternoon gives plants some protection from the midday heat. Should you have temperate winters, you can plant tender herbs and expect them to survive year-round, given normal conditions for your area.

Your climate will also largely tell you what to grow. Keep in mind that growing zones are based on the average low temperature in your area. Your zone number gives no other information about weather conditions. Some things to consider include the following:

- **Low spots** can become "frost pockets." Cold air will settle into these spots, making it likely that frost will form.
- **Excess moisture** in the form of annual rainfall and humidity is hard on the Mediterranean herbs lavender and rosemary. Too much moisture can provide a prime breeding ground for fungal diseases.
- **Lack of moisture** in the form of rain or snow can present challenges in finding water for your herbs.
- **Abundant sunshine** is necessary for plants to produce their essential oils, which give herbs their fragrance and active ingredients.
- **Frost heaves,** the heaving of the soil due to alternate freezing and thawing throughout winter months, could misplace your plants.
- **The frigid winds** of winter and, frequently, early spring can literally suck the life out of plants by drying them out.
- **Snow** can provide insulation for herbs, protecting them from cold temperatures and winds.

- **Low temperatures** will kill some tender herbs, such as rosemary and sweet marjoram. Find out how low your winter temperatures can get.
- **Drought** periods in the heat of summer should be taken into account. Herbs tolerant of dry conditions include yarrow, sage, echinacea, and thyme.

Remember that climate is not a static thing. The usual seasonal weather can abruptly change, giving you warm days when you expect cold ones, frosty days when you expect warm ones, and wet days when you expect dry ones. Try to stay flexible. Sometimes you will lose plants despite all that you do for them. Others will thrive on what I call "benign neglect." Still others will beat the odds on quirky weather changes and survive despite adverse conditions.

Microclimates

Sometimes, a small space on your property can have a different climate than your general area does. These small areas are called microclimates, and they can support a plant that has only a marginal chance given your usual conditions. Some examples of microclimates are areas sheltered from winds, land in proximity to brick walls that soak up sunlight and lend more warmth to an area, or a spot shaded by a bush or tree.

CHOOSING PLANTS

Local nurseries can be helpful about what will grow well in your area. Both chain and independent nurseries are staffed with people who like to garden and usually have experience in growing a variety of plants in your area. It is a rare gardener who doesn't like to share this information.

Take a look at other gardens to get ideas about what does well in your area. In late spring and summer months there might be garden tours sponsored by nonprofit organizations in your area. These can be a lot of fun. Take along a notebook to record specific plants that you like and want, and a camera to take pictures that will help jog your memory about some plants.

Determine your needs and what plants you wish to have in your garden. Think about how many plants you would like to grow versus how much space you have available. Grow only as many plants as you are willing to care for and use. Remember that as your interest grows, you can add to your herb collection. All of these considerations will help in making your garden plans workable, and decrease or eliminate the frustration that can come with poor planning.

Keeping a garden journal is a wonderful way to maintain a record of what plants you grow and how they do. By keeping a journal over several years you will have an ongoing report of your garden, how it fares, and what you are doing to it. Keep track of how you take care of the soil and any substances that you add to it. Notes about the weather can also be helpful in later evaluating what made your plants grow. In my journal I also like to mention when I harvest plants, and the size of the harvest I reaped.

SOIL

To me, the smell of freshly turned earth is one of the most pleasant around; it evokes feelings of new beginnings and starting life with seeds and new plants. I only smell this aroma in spring, when the weather is turning warmer and the days longer. As I drive, I find myself quickly rolling down the car window so I can smell the field that a local farmer is plowing.

Soil is not just "dirt"; it has many ingredients. Not only does soil support life in the form of the plants growing in it, but it's also a living entity in its own right. It contains water, air, and particles of rock of varying sizes. It includes dead and decaying plant and animal matter. The earth is teeming with microorganisms, insects, and earthworms, all of which contribute to the breakdown of organic matter and aeration of the soil.

Types of Soil

These are the basic soil types. You will most likely find that what you have is a combination of the following.

Clay soil is made up of the tiniest particles of rock, making it dense, heavy, and slow draining. This type of soil is challenging for gardeners; you have to be patient and wait until it is dry enough to cultivate, because it will dry out much later than other soil types. Plant roots have to struggle to penetrate it. If it is too wet when tilled, it will dry into hard rocklike clumps that are impossible to work in. Clay warms more slowly in spring than other soils, and can dry into a hard, compacted surface in summer. Adding large quantities of organic material will give clay a much more workable texture that both you and your plants like. Organic matter in the form of composted green manure will also give clay soils the ability to drain better.

Sandy soil contains the largest rock particles of all of the soil types. It feels gritty and drains rapidly. This is both a blessing and a curse, because sandy soil will be ready to cultivate early in the year, but it will not hold moisture or fertility easily. This soil can also benefit from the addition of organic material, which will improve its texture and its ability to retain moisture and nutrients.

Loam soil is what those of us with clay or sandy soils dream about! It is a mixture of the best characteristics of sand and clay with organic matter such as composted green manure added. Also, it drains well without rapidly losing moisture and fertility. Plant roots can easily grow into a loam soil. Do add organic matter periodically to enhance loam's fertility by replacing the nutrients used by the plants you grew there.

If you have soil that is difficult or impossible to work with for any reason, then it is probably easier to import some topsoil for raised beds, or buy potting mix and grow herbs in containers. Either of these can be a simple solution to difficult growing conditions.

Organic Amendments to Soil

"Feed the soil, not the plants" is a saying used by many organic farmers and gardeners. The idea is that soil is a living thing, and if it is "fed" it will in turn feed any plants grown in it. Rather than giving plants quickly absorbed chemical fertilizer mixes, give it different organic substances such as compost, rotted animal manure, or green manure, that enhance its fertility by increasing its humus content — a dark, nutrient-rich substance that gives good soil its crumbly texture and fertility. Your plants then draw up the nutrients through their roots for optimal growth. Adding organic substances to the soil supports the earthworms, small insects, and microorganisms that live there and break down plant and animal matter. This act of digesting the debris give the soil humus.

Treating the soil in this manner is a long-term investment in its quality. It may not mean much to you right now, but watching the soil gradually improve is quite gratifying and represents a positive treatment of the earth. My husband and I made a promise to leave the soil on our property better than we found it. Every season we add more compost and other organic material to our heavy clay soil. We don't have loam yet, but each season it is easier to work with, and our plants are healthier and give better yields at harvesttime.

This whole process is a cycle of life: Humus-rich soil feeds plants, and plant debris composts and feeds the soil. It is a logical way to care for the earth that nurtures us and gives us wonderful plants to use.

Composting

Adding organic material to the soil is an exercise in recycling. Many materials that you now toss into the trash and take to the landfill can be composted and worked into your garden soil.

Indeed, the best way to add organic matter to soil is by making compost. You can use many different materials gleaned from your kitchen, yard, and garden. Gathering material to be composted can be something everyone in the family can do, and it will quickly become a habit.

There are as many ways to make compost as there are gardeners. The easiest and least time consuming is to pile layers of any or all of the following ingredients up to 3 feet high. Use a pitchfork to turn and stir it if you want and have the time. Add enough water to keep the pile moist. Let the pile sit, and it will decay over several months. The size of the pile will decrease as the materials decay. The compost is ready to use when it is dark and crumbly and you can no longer recognize its individual ingredients.

Compost Ingredients

- Dried pine needles
- Grass clippings from yards that are not sprayed with herbicides or pesticides (be sure to mix with other ingredients, because grass clippings alone will compact too much to decay properly)
- Straw
- Dried leaves (if these are chopped up they will decompose more quickly)
- Sawdust from untreated lumber (not walnut or cedar)
- Vegetable and fruit peels and cores
- Coffee grounds (including unbleached coffee filter papers), and used tea bags with their contents
- Overripe fruits and vegetables
- Crushed eggshells
- Manure of any livestock animal such as cow, pig, llama, rabbit, horse, or chicken is suitable
- Weeds that have not developed seeds
- Discarded plants and produce from the garden
- Wood ashes, in small amounts
- Shredded newspaper
- Disease-free potting soil discarded from previously used containers
- Human hair trimmings

If you are concerned about weed seeds in your compost pile, place all weeds and grasses in a black plastic garbage bag and leave in the sun for 2 weeks before emptying the contents onto the pile. The heat in the bag often kills the seeds.

Do Not Add to Compost

- Sewage sludge (possibly contains heavy-metal contamination)
- Cat and dog manure (can transmit diseases)
- Human waste (can transmit diseases)

- Meat scraps (can attract pests to your compost pile)
- Fat scraps, including salad dressing oil (oils and fats become rancid)
- Diseased plants (can transmit diseases)
- Noxious weeds (seeds or roots can bring these weeds into your garden)
- Charcoal briquettes or their ashes (possibly contain petroleum-based contaminants)

Green Manure

Another way to add organic material to your soil is to plant (in fall or early spring) a green-manure cover crop, which you'll let grow for a time, then till under. Planting green-manure crops between other plants will serve to keep the soil in place, preventing erosion from water and wind. The best choice for green manure is a noninvasive grain or legume. Legume crops are nitrogen fixing — they capture nitrogen from the air, and when the plants are then tilled into the soil, the nitrogen is added to it. There it will decompose, releasing organic matter and nutrients to your soil. Wait a couple of weeks for the green manure to start decomposing before planting any crops.

If you have planted a tall-growing cover crop, it is a good idea to mow it before tilling. One season we made the mistake of tilling in buckwheat without cutting it first, and the stems kept wrapping around the tines of the tiller. Mowing will also chop up the cover crop, helping it decompose more quickly.

Green-Manure Crops

CROP	TYPE OF PLANT	WHEN TO PLANT
Alfalfa	legume	spring
White Dutch clover	legume	spring or early fall
Red clover	legume	spring or early fall
Fava beans	legume	spring
Winter vetch	legume	fall
Winter rye	grain	fall
Winter wheat	grain	fall
Buckwheat	grain	spring
Oats	grain	spring

Green-manure crops aren't just used to prepare a bed's soil, though. They can be planted among other plants in your garden to help suppress weeds. When used in this way they are called cover crops. Planting green-manure crops in empty spaces where plants have been harvested and between rows of plants will eventually return nutrients and organic matter to the fallow ground.

DETERMINING DRAINAGE AND WATER REQUIREMENTS

The amount of water available to plants is an important garden-site consideration. Water keeps the cells in plants turgid, or full and plump. It also delivers nutrients to the plant. Deep-watering is essential; watering only the surface of the soil will cause shallow root growth. While too little water can dry out your plants, too much water can "drown" a plant, encouraging fungal diseases and causing the roots to rot.

If you live in a climate with large amounts of rainfall, a planting spot with good drainage is essential. If you are trying to garden on a spot that stays wet for prolonged periods of time or has difficult to impossible soil conditions, make raised beds to grow your herbs. A hot, dry climate may call for the use of soaker hoses or drip irrigation. These two setups will deliver water right down through the surface of the soil to the root system, allowing the water to soak in deeply without evaporating. If you have soil that retains a lot of water (like clay) or soil that lets water drain quickly (like sand), add lots of organic matter.

Most of the herbs that I discuss in this book will tolerate dry to normal conditions, with the exception of peppermint and ginger. These two will grow in quite wet conditions.

Creating Raised Beds

I have mentioned raised beds frequently, so let me take some time to discuss how to make them. Raised beds must be made with soil that has an ample amount of organic matter to promote drainage and prevent settling and compaction. If you are planning raised beds with soil that does not contain lots of organic matter, you may need to import some good topsoil. Enhance any soil in your raised beds with compost, or grow a green-manure crop and dig it in.

The height of the beds can vary from 3 inches to several feet. If you plan beds higher than 8 inches, you must build a support around them. This can be made from cedar or redwood timbers, brick, concrete blocks, stone, or "logs" made from recycled plastic (available at many lumber stores).

To make a bed 3 to 8 inches high, mark off the area where you want your bed. Pull soil toward you with a rake, slanting the sides outward and downward toward the ground. Go to the opposite side of the bed and again rake soil toward you, making an outward slant on this side also. Repeat this procedure on the ends of the demarcated bed. Smooth the top of the soil with a rake before planting.

The act of pulling the topsoil into the beds will create sunken paths around them. Place a heavy layer of mulch (leaves or straw are good) on these paths to prevent compaction of the soil when it is walked on. Or you can plant a low-growing cover crop such as white Dutch clover on them.

There are many benefits to planting in raised beds. Because of the high-quality soil used to make them, you can plant more herbs in close quarters within the beds, providing a high yield in a small space. Also, their height can make it easier to garden if you cannot tolerate stooping, kneeling, or bending.

Raised beds are recommended in areas that have poor drainage.

SELECTING AND APPLYING FERTILIZER

Plants that have the proper nutrients available to them are healthier, and less susceptible to disease and pest damage. The best way to give plants the nutrients they need is to feed your soil. The plants can then take up the nutrients they need.

Too much fertilizer can be as detrimental as too little. Get soil samples from your garden and have them tested to see what your soil might need before adding fertilizers randomly. Your County Extension Service office can steer you to companies that do soil testing. Most will give you instructions and containers in which to collect your soil.

Water generously after any fertilizer is added to the soil. This will help it to become more available to the plants; in the case of organic fertilizers, it will also help them break down.

Many herbs do well in average to "lean" soil — soil that is not overly fertile. Usually good soil preparation and the addition of organic matter in the form of compost or decomposed green manure will be enough for your herb gardens to thrive.

Adjusting the pH

Your soil pH, which is one of the values given to you on a soil test, is an indication of whether your soil is acidic or alkaline. Soil pH ranges from 1 to 14; a pH of 7 is neutral, below 7 acidic, and above 7 alkaline. A pH that's too acidic or too alkaline can reduce the availability of soil nutrients to your plants. Different plants prefer acidic or alkaline soils. Most herbs do well in slightly acidic soil (pH 6.0–7.0).

Barbara Bridges and her family run Southern Perennials & Herbs in Tylertown, Mississippi, a wholesale and retail mail-order nursery for the Deep South. They're in Zone 8, which gives them summer temperatures in the high 90s F (high 30s C), mild winters with low temperatures in the teens (about –9°C), and high humidity with 50-plus inches of rain per year.

The well-drained soil of raised beds helps prevent plant rotting. Barbara says that yarrow and sage in particular have problems with rot.

Rosemary and ginger are hardy perennials for them. They have good success growing lemon balm and purple coneflower as perennials.

To meet the challenges of Zone 8 gardening, Barbara suggests planting herb gardens so that they receive afternoon shade in summer. She advises that you know which herbs do best at different times of the growing season. (See Resources for more information.)

To raise the pH of your soil, add dolomitic limestone. To lower the pH, add sulfur. The packages of each additive will give you specific directions.

Natural Fertilizers or Chemical Fertilizers?

Just as you personally need a well-balanced diet, your plants need a balance of nutrients for optimal health. Nitrogen (N) encourages the green leafy growth of plants. Phosphorus (P) plays a part in root growth and disease resistance. Potassium (K) helps in root development and good cell-wall structure. Trace elements contribute to the general good health and growth of your plants, each in its own way.

There are a lot of fertilizers on the market. Some are made from substances found in nature. Others are chemical fertilizers that are produced synthetically. All combine nitrogen, phosphorus, and/or potassium, listed on the package as N-P-K. The higher the number corresponding to each nutrient, the more of that nutrient there is. Depending on the source of the fertilizer, trace minerals may be included in its composition.

Chemical fertilizers are generally readily available to plants, giving them quick food — but doing little for the composition of the soil in the long term. They are a poor choice when your intent is to feed the soil.

On the other hand, most organic fertilizers must break down before their components are readily available to plants. It is my opinion that if you add organic matter to your soil in the form of compost and green manure, you shouldn't generally need to add many other fertilizers. Compost and green manure will provide the soil with most nutrients, and will make them available for the plants to take up as needed. A soil test will give you specific information about any further soil additions you might need.

Types of Organic Fertilizer

Organic fertilizers are made from a variety of ingredients. The following list will give you an idea of what is available.

Alfalfa meal. Made from finely ground dried alfalfa, it is high in nitrogen.

Blood meal. This is high in nitrogen and has small amounts of phosphorus and potassium. Due to its high nitrogen content, blood meal added to your compost pile will break it down more quickly. Use it sparingly in the garden — the high nitrogen content can "burn" or harm your plants.

Bonemeal. This is a natural source of phosphorus and calcium. I find that when I add this to the soil, its smell is inviting to dogs, encouraging them to dig. For this reason, use bonemeal with some caution if dogs have access to your gardens.

Cottonseed meal. This contains nitrogen plus small amounts of phosphorus and potassium. Check the source of your cottonseed meal carefully. Cotton is a crop often treated with a lot of pesticides, and the meal may have residues. Check the package for the words *certified pesticide-free*.

Greensand. This mineral mined from ancient seabeds contains potassium and trace elements. The latter are often overlooked when feeding the soil, but they are quite essential for good plant growth.

Kelp meal. This sea crop contains potassium, trace elements, and growth enhancers. Adding small amounts to the soil help "drought-proof" your plants — they'll be more tolerant of prolonged dry conditions. The growth enhancers seem to help plants take up nutrients more efficiently, but their entire action is not yet clear.

Manure. You can add manure from horses, sheep, llamas, chickens, rabbits, cows, and pigs to your garden soil. Allow the manure to decompose first, though, or the high nitrogen content can "burn" your crops.

The Benefits of Mulch

Adding a layer of mulch to your garden can accomplish several things. It can help the soil retain moisture — a boon to those in dry climates or with drought ridden summers. It also provides insulation, moderating soil temperatures despite the actual temperature fluctuations of the air. It helps prevent soil from heaving, which evicts plants from their homes by alternate freezing and thawing. It will also discourage weed growth.

Mulch serves as an anchor for the soil. You can slow and often prevent erosion by applying a layer of mulch. This is particularly important for areas prone to wind and water erosion, including wind-exposed areas and slopes into which rains and melting snows can etch gullies, stripping away valuable topsoil in the process.

The main reason I mulch is to keep down weeds. When you garden on as much space as I do without herbicides, mulch is a necessity. It prevents light, air, and moisture from getting to weed seeds, thus keeping them from sprouting.

Types of Mulch

There is a variety of mulches available. Some, such as grass clippings and compost, are free if you put in a bit of work. Commercial products like bagged chipped wood or pine bark will cost you some money.

To me, organic gardening makes sense from a long-term perspective. Organic means growing plants without the use of synthetic pesticides, herbicides, fertilizers, and/or growth additives. The potential for any of these to alter the environment and affect all living creatures in a negative way is significant.

Land stewardship — gardening practices that look to the long-term quality and preservation of the soil — is key to organic gardening. Crops are grown with a sense of balance that includes the health of the people raising and consuming the crop, as well as the earth that nurtures it. Everything and everybody involved remains unaffected by the potentially harmful substances, resulting in a healthier environment.

Leonard Brooks, Director of the Shaker Library and Shaker Museum in New Gloucester, Maine, says that the Sabbathday Lake Shaker Community there has been growing and selling herbs since 1799. Located in Zone 4, their average annual temperature is 44°F (7°C). They have 10 to 20 days of below-zero temperatures, with 50 to 70 inches of snow in winter. The rest of the year brings an annual average of 42 inches of rain.

The herb gardeners at Sabbathday Lake see a lot of winterkill and dieback of sage; they cut back dead growth in spring when the new growth appears. Maine gardeners also struggle with deer as garden pests.

Leonard's special gardening tips include harvesting plants right before they flower, and sidedressing plants with compost, rock phosphate, and bonemeal. Additionally, different varieties of mint should not be planted close to one another. (See Resources for more information.)

Organic mulches include:

Chipped wood (usually cypress or hardwood here in the Midwest) is commercially packaged. Chipped wood, which you can obtain from trimmings along roadsides and power lines, is also organic. Do not use if black walnut, cedar, poison ivy, or poison oak is contained in the mix. The people doing the trimming can tell you what kinds of wood they have chipped.

Chipped pine bark is very lightweight and can float away in heavy rains.

Pine needles are frequently used as mulch in the southern states. They smell great when stepped on.

Straw can contain a lot of weed seeds and make your weed problems worse; check with the source of your straw.

Compost can be bought commercially packaged, or you can make it yourself. To make your own, see page 71.

Grass clippings should not be used if herbicides and pesticides are applied to the grass. In addition, beware of weed seeds.

Leaves need to be chopped up to help them break down more quickly.

Newspaper, in order to be effective, must be placed in three or four layers on the ground. Use only the black-and-white sheets. If desired, you can cover the layers with other mulch materials.

Sawdust also works well. Aged sawdust has a better texture than fresh.

Synthetic mulches include:

Black plastic, which looks better covered with a natural mulch material. It prevents air, water, or nutrients from getting into the soil.

Landscape fabric has tiny holes in it to allow air, water, and nutrients to permeate its surface and go into the soil. This, too, looks better covered with a natural mulch material.

Stone is a mineral that is available in various sizes/types, and is best preceded by a layer of plastic or landscape fabric to prevent weeds from growing through.

The ideal time to lay mulch is when the soil is moist, but not waterlogged, and has been warmed by the heat of spring. I usually wait to mulch until any seeds or small plants I have planted become established, or any perennials are up and growing for the season. I lay three to four layers of newspaper, followed by 3 to 4 inches of cypress mulch or pine needles in my herb and perennial beds. My vegetable gardens get layers of newspaper followed by 5 to 6 inches of straw, which eventually settles to 4 inches.

Mulch should be applied to bare soil; any preexisting weeds must be removed. If not removed weeds will most likely grow through the mulch. Do not apply mulch to extremely wet or poorly drained soil, and also avoid applying to cold soil. If you tend to have very dry soil, water your plants well before adding mulch.

When wet, mulch can cause stems to rot. It is best to leave a 2- to 3-inch space between the edge of the mulch and the stems of the plants. This gives you space in which to "scratch in" fertilizers, and to water the soil directly as well. You can bury soaker hoses in a layer of mulch next to the plants and leave them there for the growing season; keep the connection to the soaker hoses exposed so you can hook them to a regular hose at watering time.

One of mulch's biggest drawbacks is that pests like to hide in it. If your plants become pest targets, examine the mulch thoroughly for potential hiding places. The pests may even be laying their eggs in the mulch.

Organic mulches will eventually break down and return to the soil. To do this the mulch requires nitrogen, which it takes from the soil. To prevent decaying mulch from stealing nitrogen from your plants, don't mix the mulch into the soil after you have laid it down. If you want to incorporate the mulch into the soil as an organic additive, fall is a good time to do this. This will give the mulch a chance to break down before your next growing season. Wood chip mulches will take several seasons to break down and be fully incorporated into the soil. Additional mulch can be applied around perennials, if needed, from one season to the next; the existing mulch need not be disturbed.

EDGING YOUR HERB BEDS

There is nothing much more frustrating than preparing, planting, and mulching a bed only to have the grass grow into it because it was not edged properly. Edging, which provides a natural or artificial barrier to stop the overgrowth of grass and weeds into your prepared beds, should be part of your bed preparation.

There are several ways to edge a garden; the least expensive is to use a garden spade or edger (a tool that looks like a flat half moon with a handle) to cut a 1-inch-wide and 3-inch-deep wedge of turf and soil from the edge of your bed and the edge of the lawn. This gives you a gap from which grass roots have been removed. Fill it with mulch, which acts as a natural barrier keeping grass from growing into the herb beds.

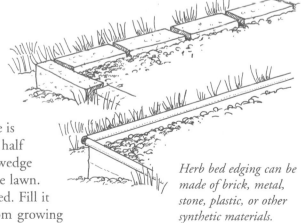

Herb bed edging can be made of brick, metal, stone, plastic, or other synthetic materials.

Teri Dunn, a gardening writer and editor, has recently written a book called *100 Favorite Herbs* (Metro Books). She gardens in the Northwestern part of the United States, an area I consider a year-round gardening mecca.

Terri pointed out that her Zone 8 conditions can present some challenges. The climate is one of extremes, with winter rains drowning tender plants and drought-like summers drying others. In addition, poor drainage can lead to rot for herbs such as sage, chamomile, and rosemary.

Herbs that like her hot, dry summers include thyme, sage, rosemary, yarrow, garlic, fennel, sweet marjoram, calendula, and purple coneflower. Peppermint often needs supplemental watering in summer. Her attempts at growing feverfew in half sun were disappointing.

Teri's special advice to gardeners in her area is "expect to win a few [and] lose a few." I think these wise words could apply to gardeners in all parts of the country.

Other physical barriers include materials such as metal edging, plastic edging, bricks, and stones. All can be placed between where the grass ends and the herb bed begins, providing a barrier that grass roots cannot grow through.

A CHECKLIST FOR PREPARING YOUR HERB BEDS

To make your herb bed preparation as smooth as possible, follow these steps:

1. Choose a site. Look at how much sunlight, drainage, and space you have, and how large a garden you are willing and able to care for.
2. Call for a utilities line search before you dig.
3. Remove existing turf by shaving it off with a flat-edged spade. Place it on your compost pile turf-side down, or move it to a bare area of your lawn with the roots down and water it to help it become established there.
4. Dig in lots of organic matter in the form of compost or green manure.
5. Have a soil sample tested for fertility and soil pH two or three weeks after digging in the organic matter.
6. Add amendments if indicated by the results of your soil test.
7. If you like, shape raised beds or (on a slope) terraces.
8. After tilling, rake the bed to break up clods of soil. Remove any rocks, roots, weeds, or grasses that didn't come away with the sod.
9. When the weather has settled and the soil is warm, plant herb seeds according to seed packet directions and water them in thoroughly. Place short sticks in the soil to mark where you have planted the seeds. Or place herb plants in the soil and water them thoroughly.
10. After the seeds have sprouted and developed a second set of leaves or the plants have shown new growth, apply mulch. If the soil is dry, water it first.

HOW LONG WILL MY HERBS LIVE?

Herbs, like other plants, are broken down into different categories depending upon their life span. Annuals are plants that live, bloom, produce seeds, and die in one season. The advantage of growing annuals is that you can plant a different variety each season in the same spot. Examples of annual herbs include calendula, cayenne, German chamomile, dill, and garlic.

Biennials are plants that grow the first year then bloom, bear seeds, and die the second year. Biennials are interesting because they give you something different each year of their life. Parsley and red clover are examples of biennials.

Perennials are plants that bloom yearly, surviving winters to return every year for several years. They also spread and multiply to give you additional plants. This category includes catnip, echinacea, fennel, feverfew, selected lavenders, lemon balm, peppermint, sage, thyme, valerian, and yarrow.

Tender perennials are not always given a category all their own, but due to the changing temperatures in many areas, I like to mention them as one. Tender perennials are plants that flower every year but will only survive winter in climates where the temperature doesn't drop to freezing. I like tender perennials despite their susceptibility to cold. They keep me company in the house in winter, where I continue to use them fresh. Aloe, ginger, sweet marjoram, and rosemary are all tender perennials.

SELECTING THE TOOLS FOR THE JOB

The market for garden tools is huge, and there are some very good tools and some very poor gimmicks available to you. Catalogs, garden stores, hardware stores, and discount stores all sell gardeners' tools and accessories. I find that looking over and handling the tools I want to purchase helps me determine their quality and suitability. Buying good-quality tools is a long-term investment — it doesn't pay to look only for the bargains when you buy garden tools. I want the kind that will hold up to the job and last for many seasons. If a bargain-priced tool fits those needs, then so much the better.

Before you spend a lot of money on gardening tools, though, assess what you need. Think about the amount of space you are planning to use for your garden. For small spaces a garden fork, rake, shovel, and edger are probably all you will need to work the soil. If you're going to plant your entire front yard, perhaps a tiller should be on your list.

Where is your water source? If it is far away from your plants, think about how you will get water to them. Measure how much hose you will need. Buy good-quality hose with brass couplings. Cheap hose will bend and kink easily, cutting off the flow of water and forcing you to waste time finding the kink every time you move it. If you live in a hot, dry climate, perhaps a soaker hose or drip irrigation equipment would be a good choice for watering. For container plantings, a gallon-sized sprinkling can comes in handy.

How do you want to carry your tools and supplies? If you are container-gardening on a patio, a good-sized bucket will hold everything. If you're tending to many beds or a large garden, you might want a wheelbarrow or garden cart.

GARDENING TOOLS

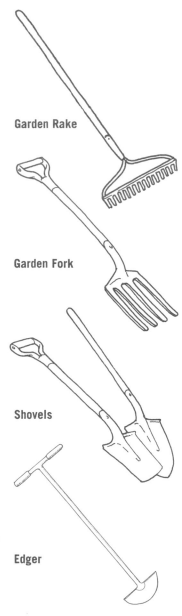

Garden Rake

Garden Fork

Shovels

Edger

Choosing tools is especially important if you have health or physical restrictions. A tool that's too heavy or bulky might not be appropriate for your level of strength. Instead, choose tools and equipment that enable you to expend a minimum of energy.

For all gardeners, a hands-on inspection when selecting tools is important. Pick up any tool that you are contemplating for purchase and hold it in your hands. Is the handle comfortable to touch? Does the tool feel well balanced? Is it too heavy for you to use for a long time? Are separate parts of the tool fastened together securely? Is it the right size for the job? Take all of these questions into consideration when purchasing your gardening equipment.

Use Your Hands

Hand tools are a must for gardening, particularly in containers and small beds. Getting down and working in among the plants is part of the process, and good tools are critical to making this job easier.

A hand trowel is an essential for me. Get a sturdy one that will hold up to repeated digging. I have found that the weak spot in many trowels is where the handle attaches to the blade. Repeated digging in heavy soil will cause this spot to bend and break. Look for a trowel that is cast all in one piece, or one sturdily welded together and made of steel or another hard metal. Good for planting and weeding, a garden trowel will become one of the tools that you never forget when heading to the garden.

A hand weeder with a pronged end is helpful. It has a long reach to dig down into the soil to cut off weed roots at a deep level, slowing their reappearance. Its small width makes it easy to get in among plants and single out weeds to remove.

A hand garden cultivator is also helpful for weeding. It looks like an extra-large fork with its tines all bent at a 90-degree angle to the handle. It is good for scratching out shallow-rooted weeds and working soil amendments in around plants. This tool also comes in handy when you're planting tiny seeds that do not need to be covered with much soil. Use the tines to scratch in the seeds, covering them lightly.

Hand pruners and scissors are needed to trim out diseased or damaged parts of a plant, for harvesting, and to thin the stems in crowded plantings. Such thinning allows air to get to the plant and dry any moisture trapped within. Do not buy bargain brands of these two tools. Buy high-quality models that will hold up to repeated use and that can be sharpened.

The Long and the Short of It

Long-handled tools such as hoes, rakes, pitchforks, and shovels should have handles long enough to keep you from bending too much when using them. Hoes and rakes especially should feel well balanced when you hold them.

Serious digging tools such as garden forks and spades have shorter handles and usually a D-shaped or T-shaped handle. Make sure that the wooden handle is well anchored to the digging part of the tool and look for sturdiness at this point, because this is where the stress of the work will be. I find a garden fork indispensable. Use it for digging in soil amendments, loosening soil, and digging up plants and weeds.

Other Equipment

If you are on a limited budget, consider renting higher-priced items such as tillers and chipper/shredders. These pieces of equipment are not used frequently, and can be obtained at rental companies. If you need one during peak season, call ahead to reserve it; this will save you the frustration of having the time to do a task, but not the equipment. I also find that this is a good way to try different types of power equipment to see what I'd really like to buy.

GARDENING CLOTHES AND ACCESSORIES

Your gardening clothes should be comfortable. You should be able to move in them without binding or undue tightness, but they should not be loose enough to get caught in power equipment. Long sleeves and long-legged pants will protect you from the sun as well as from scratchy weeds and branches. A hat will also protect your face from the sun. Sturdy shoes that support your feet are a good idea, too. Gardening does not have to be a fashion show. I usually wear my older clothes to garden in because I get down on the ground and really dig into the job, resulting in very dirty and hardworked clothes.

To my way of thinking, good gardening gloves are an investment. Many kinds are available in different materials. Leather gloves are quite protective and hold up to a lot of hard use; for this reason they are my favorite kind. Rubber- or vinyl-coated models are nice to protect your hands from wet and cold conditions in early spring, but they're not well enough ventilated for warmer weather. When it comes to hard work, cloth and knit gloves wear out quickly and do little to protect your hands.

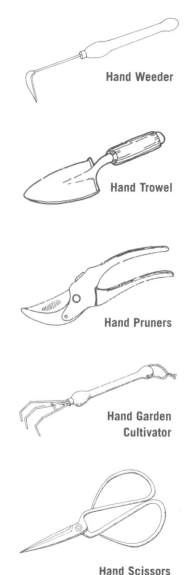

HAND TOOLS

Hand Weeder

Hand Trowel

Hand Pruners

Hand Garden Cultivator

Hand Scissors

Gardening is hard on my knees. When I get tired of squatting or bending in the garden, I inevitably end up working among my plants on my knees. This is where kneeling pads or wearable knee pads come in handy. Kneeling pads are made of dense foam rubber and cushion you from the hard ground. Some come with frames fitted with handles that are easier to get up from, and can be turned over to create a padded seat. If you are prone to leaving your pad behind as you move through the garden and still want knee protection, perhaps wearable knee pads are for you. These are usually made from a dense foam with a hardened plastic outer coating and are strapped onto your knees.

Other Accessories to Consider

Sun exposure has become a concern with the increased occurrence of skin cancers these days. Apply a layer of sunscreen to your exposed skin 20 minutes before you go outside so that it soaks in; reapply as you sweat. You may need insect repellent, too, especially in the evening when mosquitoes come out to feed. Sunglasses will help to reduce the glare and block potentially damaging UV rays from your eyes.

Special hand care is essential for gardeners. Consider applying a moisturizing hand oil or cream before going out to garden. When coming in, clean your hands by applying a layer of oil, rubbing it in, then wiping it off with a clean paper towel. Make some special skin oil by infusing herbs into the oil. (See page 12.) Make some skin salve from the herbal infused oil as well. (See page 14.) Lavender and/or calendula are good choices of herbs to use in an oil or salve.

CARING FOR TOOLS

Bring tools inside when you are finished using them for the day. Constant exposure to the elements will cause metal to rust and wood to rot, which shortens the life span of a good tool. Scrape off excess soil and plunge the metal parts into a bucket full of sand that you've mixed with 2 to 3 cups of vegetable oil to protect from rust. Wooden handles should have rough spots lightly sanded as needed to prevent splinters.

To keep all pruners and scissors clean and free from disease-carrying organisms, wipe the blades after each use with a rag dipped in rubbing alcohol. Let them air-dry before storing or using again.

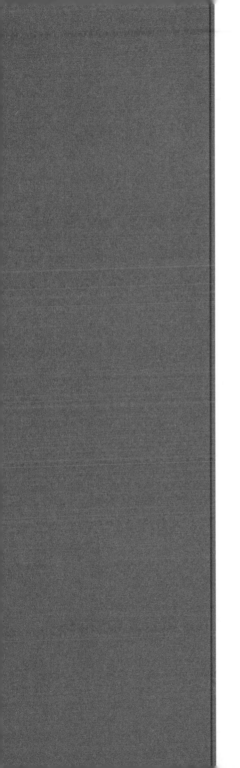

CHAPTER 5

Designing a Garden for Your Special Needs

ach of the gardens in this section has herbs specially selected for different needs. Should you have any particular minor ailments, I have grouped herbs together that can assist you in treating them. If you grow these specific herbs, you will have them readily available for use. Having one of these special gardens will help you become familiar with each of its herbs, as well as providing you with visual pleasure, aroma, and usefulness.

If you have children in your household, a Children's Herb Garden or First-Aid Garden might be a good choice. If you have trouble sleeping, the Relaxation Garden could be what you need. Evaluate your needs and those of your family. If you have the space, plant more than one of these theme gardens; you could then make connecting paths of brick, gravel, or mulch to travel from one bed to another.

I have noticed that many suburban homes today have little planted in their front yards but grass. People do not seem to enjoy or use their front yards, either. So, what better place to plant some of these herb gardens than your front yard? You'll be able to see the plants from the front windows of your home, and make an underutilized space productive. Many of these plants could also be arranged in beds next to your front or back door, for easy access and enjoyment.

If you're planting more than one of these gardens, design them to wind around your property in a deliberate path. Some of the gardens contain the same individual herbs; use these plants to connect and blend your different gardens together. That way you could take a pleasant walk around your gardens and house with your eyes moving from one group of herbs to the next, stopping to smell the plants and even taste them when appropriate.

None of these garden plans is absolute. Use your imagination and whatever plants, space, and accessories you actually have to create variations. Gardening should be flexible and not frustrate you with plans that use plants, containers, and/or space you don't have and can't obtain! The only requirement of these herbs is to be grown in areas with partial to full sun. Most of these plants — with the exception of mint — will not tolerate full shade.

For convenience, I have included in my plans the ideal numbers of plants to have available for immediate use; some of the gardens include enough extra to harvest and store for later use. These plant numbers can be increased or decreased according to which herbs you use the most and how much space you have.

Certain herbs seem to be individually suited to people. As you try different plants for different ailments, you will find some that stand out as favorites for you and your family. On the other hand, you may also try some plants that do not like your climate or gardening conditions no matter what you do. There may also be herbs you do not like for other reasons. After you discover the pros and cons of these plants, you may want to alter the herbs that you keep regularly in your gardens.

CHOOSING YOUR GARDEN

This chapter contains plans for 20 gardens tailored to meet special health needs. Choose which garden is best for you and your family, follow the instructions for growing, and be creative! Your garden is a place of enjoyment, where you can grow healing herbs to use for a variety of home remedies.

- Bath Garden
- Children's Herb Garden
- Cold and Flu Garden
- Decongestant Garden
- Eye Care Garden
- First-Aid Garden
- Hair Care Garden
- Headache Relief Garden
- Healthy Heart Garden
- Mouth Care Garden

- Rejuvenation Garden
- Relaxation Garden
- Skin Care Garden
- Sore Muscle Care Garden
- Throat Care Garden
- Traveler's Herb Garden
- Tummy Care Garden
- Woman's Care Garden
- Windowsill Medicine Cabinet

SCRATCH AND SNIFF?

I frequently mention the aroma of herbs, and how working among them and touching them is a fragrant pleasure. Each particular aroma is captured in the plant within tiny oil glands located in the leaves, flowers, or roots. Rubbing or brushing up against these plants will break open these glands. This action will release the oils and make the aroma available to you.

Bath Garden

This garden contains herbs appropriate to use in your bath. A bonus is that you can pick the herbs you would like to use for a cleansing, fragrant soak after gardening chores! The choice of mints in this garden is up to you; any mint but pennyroyal can be used in the bath. There are many types of mint, so plant the type that has the most appealing aroma to you.

CONTAINER GARDEN

The container bath garden uses various-sized containers arranged in a way that is pleasing to the eye and accommodates the space you have available. The staggered container plantings of different widths and heights lend interest. The two largest containers must be 18 inches in diameter or larger.

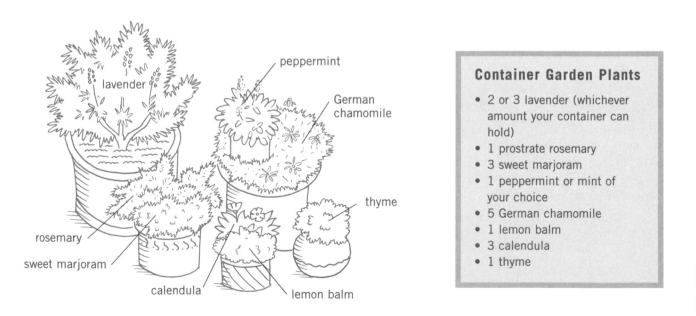

Container Garden Plants

- 2 or 3 lavender (whichever amount your container can hold)
- 1 prostrate rosemary
- 3 sweet marjoram
- 1 peppermint or mint of your choice
- 5 German chamomile
- 1 lemon balm
- 3 calendula
- 1 thyme

PLOT GARDEN

A birdbath makes an interesting visual centerpiece for this garden that enhances its theme. A fountain or classical statuary could also be placed in the center. Divide each planting with a layer of plastic or newspaper, then cover that layer with mulch, decorative stone, or brick. Other ideas include an old bathtub planted with herbs, or herbs planted along a path leading to a small pool and/or fountain.

Don't be cavalier about planting the mint in this garden. If not kept in check, it will take over and choke out the other plants. To slow this invasive tendency, plant the mint in a large container sunk into the ground. It will still want to grow over the edge of the sunken container, but it can be controlled more easily. Or you can control the mint by chopping it out from around the edges of the clump with a shovel or spade. These thinned plants can be discarded, transplanted elsewhere, given away, or divided and planted in small pots to sell.

Plot Garden Plants

- 7 lavender
- 2 peppermint or other mint
- 12 German chamomile
- 2 lemon balm
- 3 thyme
- 12 calendula
- 1 or 2 rosemary
- 7 sweet marjoram

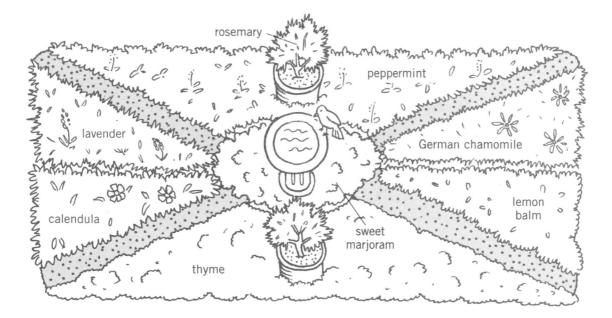

BATH RECIPES

These recipes benefit not only your skin but also your emotions by providing you with some herbal aromas to inhale as you soak away the cares of the day. Before incorporating any of these infusions into your bathwater, use the patch test on your skin. (See page 10.) If you don't take baths, follow the instructions for any of the bath mixtures and use the cooled infusion as a body splash during your shower. Use the bath bag of herbs as a washcloth.

Troubled Skin Bath

Summer can cause a variety of irritations to your skin. Try soaking in the Troubled Skin Bath as an aid in relieving some of them.

> ¼ cup fresh or 2 tablespoons dried thyme
> ¼ cup fresh or 2 tablespoons dried calendula blossoms
> 1 quart boiling water

Add the herbs to the boiling water and simmer, covered, for 10 minutes. Remove the infusion from the heat and let it cool to lukewarm. Strain the infusion and add to your bathwater.

Deodorizing Bath

All of the herbs in this recipe contain ingredients that will deodorize your body. It is a wonderful herbal mixture to enjoy after a hot day of working in the garden.

> ¼ cup fresh or 2 tablespoons dried thyme
> ¼ cup fresh or 2 tablespoons dried lavender buds
> ¼ cup fresh or 2 tablespoons dried rosemary
> 1 muslin bath bag
> 1 quart boiling water

Add the fresh or dried herbs to the bag and close snugly. Add the bag to the water and simmer, covered, for 15 minutes. Remove the infusion from the heat and cool to lukewarm. Add the infusion and bag to your bathwater, using the bag of herbs as a washcloth.

Fragrant Bath

The herbs in this recipe will give you a fresh, pleasantly scented bath.

- ¼ cup fresh or 2 tablespoons dried sweet marjoram
- 2 tablespoons fresh or 1 tablespoon dried lavender buds
- 2 tablespoons fresh or 1 tablespoon dried peppermint
- 1 muslin bath bag
- 1 quart boiling water

Add the fresh or dried herbs to the muslin bag and close snugly. Infuse the bath bag of herbs in the boiling water and simmer, covered, for 15 to 20 minutes. Let the infusion cool to lukewarm, then add it and the bath bag to your bathwater.

Relaxation Bath

- ½ cup fresh or ¼ cup dried lemon balm
- ½ cup fresh or ¼ cup dried German chamomile blossoms
- 2 cups boiling water

Add the herbs to the boiling water. Cover and infuse for 20 minutes. Strain and add to your bathwater.

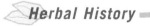

Herbal History

- Lavender came to Great Britain circa 1500 from southern France. Workers who harvested lavender flowers in the field received extra money as "hazard pay" because of the risk of being stung by bees.
- Folklore says that rosemary grows and thrives only in the house where the woman rules.

Children's Herb Garden

The Children's Herb Garden can be a magical hideaway for the child who keeps company with your garden. Give your child some of the decision-making responsibilities for designing the garden, and have him or her help plant the herbs and place the statuary and bird feeder. Because of his or her involvement, the garden will truly belong to the child.

CONTAINER GARDEN

For your container plantings, stair-step planting troughs and place them on concrete cinder blocks. Notice that dill replaces fennel in this plan. Fennel is too large for container plantings; dill and fennel share many of the same properties.

Have your child become involved in the design process by decorating the sides of the containers with brightly colored acrylic paints. Use large containers that are wide enough so that they won't tip over and injure the child. The bottoms of the containers can be weighted with stones or bricks to provide more stability. Stagger the plants according to height for greater visual interest. Plant the chickweed in a container in front of the troughs, or in the ground next to them. Place whimsical planting stakes or markers in among the plants. Get your child a small watering can so that he or she will have the responsibility of watering the plants. You can also place a Children's Herb Garden in an old red wagon or baby buggy.

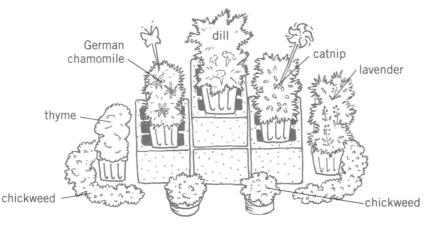

German chamomile

dill

catnip

lavender

thyme

chickweed

chickweed

Container Garden Plants

- 6 dill
- 5 German chamomile
- 3 catnip
- 5 lavender
- 5 thyme
- 4 chickweed

PLOT GARDEN

The tall fennel fence gives fragrant privacy. Little statues tucked among the herbs add interest and a nice surprise for young eyes. The inclusion of a bird feeder brings the experience of bird-watching to the garden. The bench or sandbox gives the child a reason to linger among the lavender plants. An alternative seating idea is to place a large flat stone for the child to sit upon. For extra fun, plant a "fennel forest" with mazelike paths through it.

Plant as many fennel plants as it takes to cover the perimeter of the area. If chickweed doesn't grow naturally in your cultivated soil, as it so often does, transplant it from a part of your garden where it is unwelcome. Let the chickweed spread in a 2-foot by 1-foot area. Birds are attracted to the seeds of the chickweed plant, giving your child another opportunity to enjoy bird-watching.

Plot Garden Plants

- 18–24 German chamomile
- 5 catnip
- 12 lavender
- 1 ginger rhizome in a container
- 7 thyme
- 19–20 fennel
- 5–6 chickweed

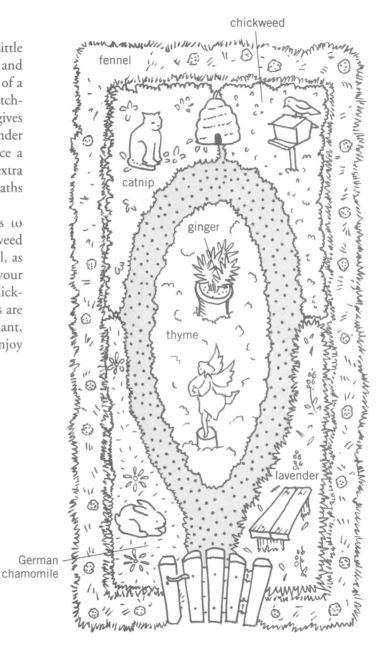

CHILDREN'S RECIPES

Adding some simple herbal treatments to your childcare regimen will benefit both of you. You will have the satisfaction of preparing natural treatments from your herbal bounty, and your child will learn about the usefulness of different plants.

Naptime Pillow

This herbal mix could be put into an animal-shaped pillow to make it more special for the child.

> 1 6-inch-square empty pillowcase
> Equal amounts dried lavender and dried chamomile blossoms

If you don't have a premade pillowcase, fold a piece of fabric or a washcloth in half and sew three sides shut. Have the child fill the pillow with the lavender and chamomile blossoms, and then sew up the open end. Place the naptime pillow between the bed pillow and pillowcase, and let the child sleep on it for a fragrant nap.

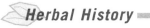 **Herbal History**

- Anglo Saxons of old drank fennel tea to lessen hunger pangs during the fasting period of Lent.
- In Hungary, oil of chamomile is distilled and included as an ingredient in the process used to coat glass and porcelain.

A Tasty Remedy

I started making candied ginger for our son to have available if he has an upset stomach. This recipe is an ongoing 4-day project, so plan to be around your kitchen for an hour or so each day during the process. These will store indefinitely and are quite tasty; they can be used as an after-dinner treat as well as for stomach upsets.

- 2 cups peeled fresh ginger cut into ½-inch squares
- 1 cup sugar, divided
- ½ lemon or orange, peeled and sliced thinly
- 1 cup light corn syrup

1. Place the ginger in a saucepan and cover with water. Put on the lid and slowly bring to a boil. Simmer until the pieces of ginger are tender when pierced with a fork. Remove from heat. Keep covered and let the mixture sit overnight at room temperature.
2. The next day, bring the mixture to a boil, then reduce the heat and simmer for 15 minutes. Add the lemon or orange slices and corn syrup. Simmer uncovered for 15 minutes longer, stirring occasionally. Remove the pan from the heat, keep covered, and again let stand overnight.
3. The following day, bring the mixture to a boil. Stir in ½ cup of the sugar, bring to a boil again, then simmer uncovered for 30 minutes. Stir in the remaining ½ cup sugar and bring to a boil, then remove from heat. Cover and let stand overnight.
4. Bring to a boil once again. When the ginger is translucent and the syrup drops heavily from the side of a spoon, remove the ginger from the syrup. (Save the syrup for use as a remedy in itself, or as a surprise flavor on pancakes.) Dry the ginger on a wire rack with foil or waxed paper under it overnight or longer. When the ginger is dry (it will still feel tacky), dust it with granulated sugar and store in a tightly covered jar.

NATURAL FOOD STORE NOTES

Nancy Kirklin, the owner and proprietor of Franklin Cornucopia in Franklin, Indiana, says that some customers use ginger to help cleanse their systems through perspiration.

Cold and Flu Garden

When cooler winter weather arrives here in Indiana colds and flus often arrive, too. Raise one of these gardens for an herbal harvest that can be used to treat your cold or flu.

PLOT GARDEN #1

A smaller garden for these plants could be tiered or terraced, bordered on two sides by yarrow and echinacea. Plant prostrate rosemary on the bottom row so that it will spill over the edge. Use flat stones stacked on top of each other or cedar logs to support the soil in each tier. Do not use treated lumber, because the chemicals used in treating the wood can leach into the soil and subsequently be absorbed into the herbs.

For some added character, try placing an old wooden ladder or wagon wheel on your prepared ground. Plant different herbs between the spokes or rungs.

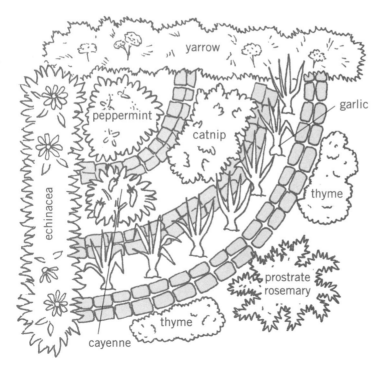

Plants for Plot Garden #1

- 1 peppermint
- 1 catnip
- 1 cayenne pepper
- 5 garlic cloves
- 2 thyme
- 1 prostrate rosemary
- 2 yarrow
- 3 echinacea

PLOT GARDEN #2

This plan can take up quite a large space. Plant a patchwork quilt of herbs of differing heights, colors, and textures. Remember that the peppermint can become invasive with very little encouragement. To slow it, plant it in a large tub or container with holes in the bottom for drainage and sink it into the ground. Butterflies will be drawn to the echinacea and yarrow.

Plants for Plot Garden #2

- 4 thyme
- 9 garlic cloves
- 3 cayenne pepper
- 1 yarrow
- 2 echinacea
- 1 peppermint
- 2 rosemary

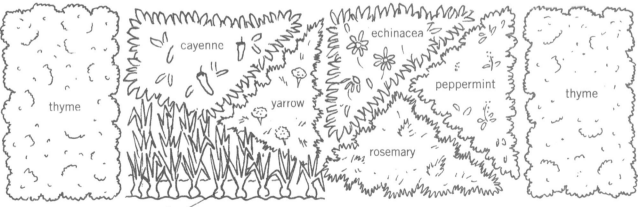

COLD AND FLU RECIPES

Most people have trouble avoiding a cold or flu, especially in the winter. These recipes will provide you with herbal comfort when you're ill.

Herbal Broth

Flavorful, warming, and packed with vitamins, this broth can be sipped easily from a mug.

- 6 minced garlic cloves
- 1 tablespoon olive oil
- 2 cups water or vegetable broth
- 1 teaspoon fine-chopped fresh cayenne pepper, or ½ teaspoon dried powdered cayenne
- 1 teaspoon fine-chopped fresh or ½ teaspoon dried rosemary
- ½ teaspoon fresh or ¼ teaspoon dried thyme
- Pinch to ¼ teaspoon salt, to taste, if the vegetable broth is unsalted

Add the garlic to the olive oil and sauté over high heat briefly, until the garlic starts to change color. Add the broth or water, turn the heat down to medium-low, and simmer for 20 minutes. Add all of the herbs and salt to taste. Simmer for 5 more minutes, then serve. Sip slowly.

Herbal Inhaler

The aromas from this herbal infusion will aid in clearing your stuffy nose.

- 2 quarts water
- ¼ cup fresh or 2 tablespoons dried yarrow
- ¼ cup fresh or 2 tablespoons dried peppermint
- 1 tablespoon fresh or 2 teaspoons dried rosemary
- 1 tablespoon fresh or 2 teaspoons dried thyme

Place the water in a saucepan on the stove. Add all of the herbs. Simmer uncovered over low heat for 30 to 45 minutes. This allows the herbal essences to drift through the house. Do not allow the pan's contents to boil dry.

To simmer these herbs without having to keep as close an eye on them, place the herbs and hot water in a slow cooker. Leave it uncovered and set on high. This can be left unsupervised for an hour or two.

Peppermint Inhalation

When suffering from congestion due to colds and/or sinus conditions, peppermint can be helpful simmered in water as an inhalation.

½ cup dried or 1 cup fresh peppermint
1 quart boiling water

Add water and peppermint to an enamel or stainless-steel saucepan. Allow this mixture to simmer uncovered on the stovetop, this will release the peppermint aroma into the air. You will enjoy greater benefits if you are in the same room as the mixture.

An alternative way to prepare the inhalation is in a small simmering potpourri pot, which is more portable and can be placed in any room you choose. Do not allow the mixture to boil dry; add more water if needed.

Thyme-Infused Honey

This is a most pleasant way to ingest thyme when you're suffering from a cold and congestion.

1 cup honey
½ cup fresh or ¼ cup dried thyme

Combine the two ingredients and heat gently over low heat for 15 to 20 minutes, making sure the honey does not boil or scorch. Remove from the heat and allow the honey to cool. Strain out the herbs, then bottle the honey and label it. To relieve colds, coughs, and sore throats, take 1 teaspoon of honey three times a day. You can also add a teaspoon to a cup of regular hot tea and sip slowly.

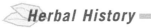

Herbal History

- Yarrow has been called staunch weed and noseblod because of its ability to stop bleeding.
- In early colonial days in Jamaica, hot pepper juice was placed in slaves' eyes as a means of punishment.
- The French served catnip tea to guests before bedtime to help settle their stomachs.

Decongestant Garden

Grow these herbs if you are prone to sinus problems, allergies, and/or colds. You can grow yarrow, catnip, and cayenne in a relatively small space. The containers of ginger and rosemary stand as sentinels over the rest of the garden.

PLOT GARDEN

Plant the yarrow, catnip, and cayenne in the ground. Place containers of ginger and rosemary on pedestals of different heights for a unique look.

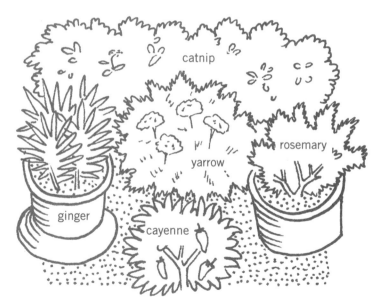

Plot Garden Plants

- 1 ginger rhizome
- 1 rosemary
- 2 yarrow
- 2 catnip
- 1 cayenne

CONTAINER GARDEN

A grouping of various containers in sizes appropriate for your plants and different enough for an interesting contrast is a good choice for these herbs. Such an arrangement would look attractive in the corner of a patio or deck.

To make your rosemary plant into a standard, plant it in a container large enough to give it room to grow. Common rosemary *(Rosmarinus officinalis)* is the best choice for this project. Choose a sturdy-looking central branch of the plant for the main branch or trunk of the standard, and clip the side branches and shoots from it. Furnish support in the form of a stake to keep the plant in an upright position as it grows. Clip the top growth into the shape you desire. Usually, a circular or mounded shape is easiest. As the top grows, trim or pinch back the new growth to encourage bushiness. Please note that rosemary is not a fast-growing plant; time and patience are required for success.

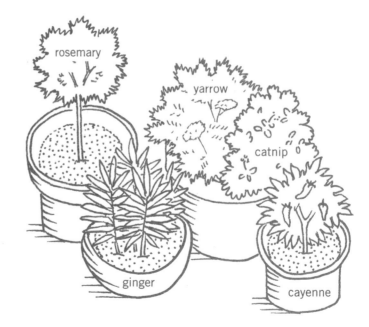

Container Garden Plants

- 1 rosemary
- 1 yarrow
- 1 catnip
- 1 ginger rhizome
- 1 cayenne

DECONGESTANT RECIPES

The feeling of stuffiness can be the most aggravating symptom of colds, allergies, and sinus problems. These herbal preparations will give you some relief.

Decongestant Inhalant

This versatile mixture is for external use only. Simmer it in a pan or place it in a reusable muslin bag for the same soothing effect.

> Equal parts dried yarrow, dried catnip, and dried rosemary
> Eucalyptus essential oil
> 1 muslin tea bag

Mix the herbs together. For each cup of dried mixture, add 4 or 5 drops of eucalyptus essential oil, if it is available. Place the mixture in a muslin tea bag. Occasionally squeeze and bring this bag close to your nose to inhale; this will relieve congestion. You also can place the bag on a warm register or in a sunny window to distribute the aroma into the air.

Or, put ¼ to ½ cup of the mixture in 1 quart of simmering water in a noncorrosive pan and let the aroma drift through your house.

When you're traveling, place the muslin bag on the dashboard of your car. The heat from the sun and the defroster will help disperse the aroma.

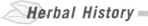 **Herbal History**

- Essential oil of rosemary is a common ingredient in cologne.
- Hunters used to stuff their cleaned game with rosemary to keep it from spoiling.
- Ginger is a common ingredient in Ayurvedic medicine preparations.

Dual-Purpose Stir Fry

Have some of this recipe to please your palate and help give you relief from congestion. This can be served as a side dish or over rice for a vegetarian main course. You don't have to be congested to enjoy this recipe!

6 cups cabbage cut into ¼-inch slices
1 tablespoon fresh ginger, grated
¼ cup water
Pinch cayenne
Pinch salt

Spray a frying pan or sauté pan with nonstick cooking spray, or coat the surface with about 1 teaspoon of vegetable oil. Place the pan on your stovetop over high heat; add the cabbage and ginger. Fry the cabbage in the oil for a couple of minutes, stirring frequently. Pour the water over the cabbage. Stir and cook the cabbage until it is crisp-tender, 10 to 15 minutes. Turn the stovetop heat down to medium-low. Add the cayenne and salt; stir the seasonings into the cabbage. Serve immediately.

Rosemary-Ginger Tea

Here is something warm and aromatic for you to sip while you lounge around recuperating.

1 tablespoon ginger, grated
1 teaspoon dried rosemary, or 2 teaspoons fresh
1 cup water

In a saucepan, heat water to boiling. Pour the boiling water over the ginger and rosemary. Cover the mixture and let it steep for 5 minutes. Strain, and pan into a mug. If desired, add up to ½ teaspoon of honey. Sip slowly.

CULINARY RELIEF

Cayenne added to any dish will give you extra vitamin C. The volatile oils in cayenne will help open your sinus passages.

Eye Care Garden

*T*he brightly colored annual blooms of calendula and chamomile show off separately in each of this garden's circles, with an intermingling of colors and plants where the circles intersect. Both plants will bloom best in the cooler temperatures of early summer and early fall. Harvesting the blooms will encourage the calendula to bloom more. German chamomile plants will wither and die in the summer heat, but self-seeded new plants will sprout and bloom as late summer cools into early fall.

CONTAINER GARDEN

A half whiskey barrel or large urn makes a good container for German chamomile and calendula. Alternately fill the container with calendula and German chamomile. Add moss to the surface of the container under the plants, or underplant with a low-growing decorative flowering thyme such as red creeping thyme or white creeping thyme. A small statue of a frog or other animal would be charming peeking out from under the herbs.

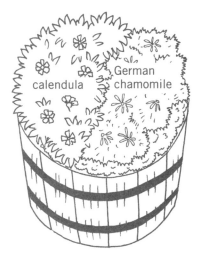

calendula

German chamomile

Container Garden Plants

- 7–8 calendula
- 7–8 German chamomile

PLOT GARDEN

Plant two intersecting circular beds. Fill one circle with calendula plants, the other with German chamomile plants. (You may need more plants than listed, depending upon the size of your prepared bed.) Fill the area where the circles intersect with alternating plantings of calendula and German chamomile.

You may want to plant the German chamomile side of the bed with a low-growing thyme such as mother of thyme, red creeping thyme, or white creeping thyme. The German chamomile will grow through the thyme plants, and the bed will have something growing in it when the German chamomile withers in the heat of summer. This is called underplanting, and is done frequently when taller plants need something growing at their base. Outline the outer perimeter of the bed with brick.

Another idea is to fill a section of a large log that has been hollowed out with soilless potting mix for planting. Alternate German chamomile and calendula plants in the log. Plant them as you would in any container. Or, plant concentric circles of German chamomile and calendula until you reach a "bull's-eye" in the center.

> ### Plot Garden Plants
> - 7–8 calendula
> - 9–12 German chamomile

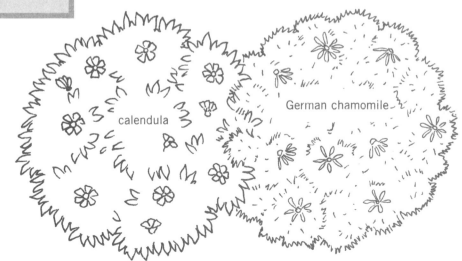

calendula

German chamomile

EYE CARE RECIPES

Some days all of your activities make your eyes tired. Relax with a pair of these eye pads on your lids and you'll feel better in less than 30 minutes.

Herb-Soaked Eye Pads

These are simple and can help to refresh your tired eyes after a busy day. Remember to do a patch test on your skin first. (See page 10.)

- 2 teaspoons dried chamomile blossoms or dried calendula blossoms
- 1 cup water
- 1 washcloth or small cotton pads

Simmer the dried chamomile blossoms or dried calendula blossoms in the water for 10 minutes. Allow to cool completely. Strain out the herbs. Dip a clean washcloth or small cotton pads into the infusion and wring out the excess water. Place the cloth or pads on your closed eyes and rest for 20 minutes.

Herbal History

- Calendula flower conserve (a preparation similar to jam) was used in colonial America as a heart medicine.
- In Brittany, it was believed that if a maiden touched calendula flowers with her bare feet she would forever be able to understand the language of birds.
- According to Shatoiya de la Tour of Dry Creek Herb Farm in Auburn, California, monks of old lay recuperating patients on large beds of Roman chamomile to soothe them.

Easy Eye Pads

The only preparation for this eye refresher is opening a box of chamomile tea bags.

> 2 chamomile tea bags
> 1 cup boiling water

Pour the boiling water over the tea bags. Leave the bags in the water until the temperature has cooled. Remove the tea bags from the water and squeeze out the excess fluid. Place one tea bag on each closed eye. Keep the teabags in place for 10 to 15 minutes. Do not discard the chamomile infusion; store it in the refrigerator and use it the next morning as an after-shower hair rinse or facial rinse.

WATCH OUT!

Your eyesight is extremely valuable. Consult with a health-care professional if you experience any of the following:

- disturbances in vision, including blurriness or double vision
- burning and/or itching of the eyes that doesn't go away
- redness of the eyes that doesn't go away
- unusual drainage or discharge from the eyes

First-Aid Garden

If you have wild plants growing on your property, you may only need to plant calendula and add a pot of aloe for your First-Aid Garden. Yarrow, plantain, and chickweed are wild plants that you can frequently find growing on their own. Chickweed is commonly found in areas where the soil has been disturbed by tilling or other means. Yarrow can be found in sunny, dry areas and does not mind being transplanted as long as the new spot receives lot of sun and good drainage. Plantain is found just about anywhere that hasn't been sprayed by herbicides.

CONTAINER GARDEN #1

Plant a 1-foot by 2-foot trough with yarrow, calendula, and aloe. Let plantain and chickweed grow in front of the trough. If you would like to grow this garden on a patio or deck, plant a second container with chickweed and plantain gathered from your yard.

For a first-aid kit on wheels, plant a First-Aid Garden in an old wagon or wheelbarrow.

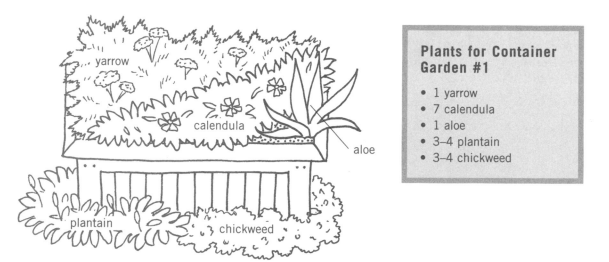

Plants for Container Garden #1

- 1 yarrow
- 7 calendula
- 1 aloe
- 3–4 plantain
- 3–4 chickweed

CONTAINER GARDEN #2

Try this design idea: Plant this garden near any other gardens or near the door of your house for the availability of quick first aid. Stagger the heights of the plants; yarrow is the tallest and should be in back. Plant the yarrow, calendula, and aloe in containers, and let the plantain and chickweed grow in the ground in front of them. Chickweed, yarrow, and plantain can be moved from elsewhere on your yard and property.

Plants for Container Garden #2

- 1 yarrow
- 4 calendula
- 1 aloe
- 4–6 plantain
- 4–6 chickweed

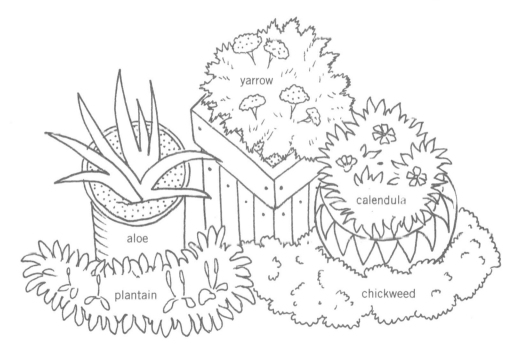

FIRST-AID RECIPES

First aid will be just outside your door with this garden and its suggested recipes.

Itch Relief Infusion

For itchy skin from any number of causes, try this infusion.

- ½ cup fresh or ¼ cup dried chickweed
- 1 cup boiling water

Infuse the chickweed in the boiling water for 10 minutes. Strain, and cool the infusion in the refrigerator. Use the infusion as a lotion on affected areas of your skin. For long term storage, pour it into ice cube trays and freeze. Store these cubes in a labeled resealable plastic bag in the freezer, removing them as needed to rub on itchy areas of the skin.

For enhanced itch relief, add the infusion to 2 tablespoons of oatmeal and allow it to soak for a few minutes. Strain, and apply as a lotion.

Cuts and Scrapes Infusion

The antibacterial properties in calendula make it an appropriate treatment for minor cuts and scrapes. As an alternative to the Cuts and Scrapes Infusion, apply fresh aloe vera gel to minor cuts and scrapes.

- 1 tablespoon dried or 2 tablespoons fresh calendula blossoms
- 1 cup boiling water

Add the calendula blossoms to the boiling water. Cover and let steep for 15 minutes, then cool to lukewarm. Apply to minor cuts and scrapes to clean them and promote healing.

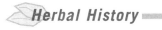

Herbal History

- In India, the Buddhists believe that calendula is sacred.
- In Mexico, calendula symbolizes death.
- Chickweed plants provide fresh seeds for birds in winter.

Insect Bite Relief

A crushed plantain leaf is a soothing remedy for an insect bite or sting. If the insect's stinger is left in (such as with a honeybee sting), first gently scrape it out of the skin using your fingernail or a dull knife edge. Then rub on the crushed leaf.

1 plantain leaf, crushed

Apply the crushed plantain leaf to the bite or sting, rubbing gently.

Minor Burn Relief

For relief of minor sunburn or other burns, apply the gel from an aloe vera leaf to the affected area.

1 aloe vera leaf, cut

Gently apply the aloe vera gel to the burn. Reapply every two hours as needed to relieve redness and discomfort.

NATURAL FOOD STORE NOTES

Chuck Landon, DaHOM, DN, PhD, who owns and operates Nature's Cupboard in Greenwood, Indiana, finds that his customers seek out calendula in a cream base to use externally for skin rashes, sunburn, and diaper rash. He finds that people like calendula cream because it is nonirritating. Internally, some of his female customers take calendula to help regulate their menstrual cycles.

Hair Care Garden

Long before there were fancy hair-care products, women used herbs to care for their hair and enhance its appearance. By growing and using this garden you will be following their lead.

CONTAINER GARDEN

Plant the herbs in a large strawberry jar. Fill the jar with potting mix, adding the plants as the mix reaches the level of each pocket. For easier watering, place a 1- to 2-inch-diameter plastic pipe with holes drilled near the level of each pocket vertically; fill in potting mix around (but not in) the pipe.

Herbs in a strawberry jar will most likely need to be treated as annuals; the pockets don't allow enough space for each plant to thrive for more than one growing season. Plant prostrate rosemary around the base, and place a sturdy upside-down saucer on the ground for the strawberry jar to sit on for added height. Plant yarrow in the top of the jar, and sage, German chamomile, and calendula in the pockets. Add more plants if you have more pockets to fill.

Bury an old double sink up to its rim in the ground and plant herbs in it for a creative look. Herbs can also be planted in old buckets or basins with multiple holes punched in the bottom for drainage.

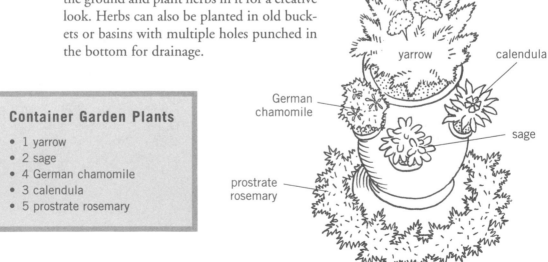

yarrow

calendula

German chamomile

sage

prostrate rosemary

Container Garden Plants

- 1 yarrow
- 2 sage
- 4 German chamomile
- 3 calendula
- 5 prostrate rosemary

PLOT GARDEN

Yarrow will become the tall focal center of this bed. Plant a shorter or dwarf variety of calendula for the border; a tall variety might overwhelm the view of the sage and rosemary plants. Use more or fewer chamomile and calendula plants than listed, depending on how many it takes for you to plant alternately as a border. The colors of the flowers lend a bright note to this garden. The more calendula blossoms you harvest, the more the plants are encouraged to bloom.

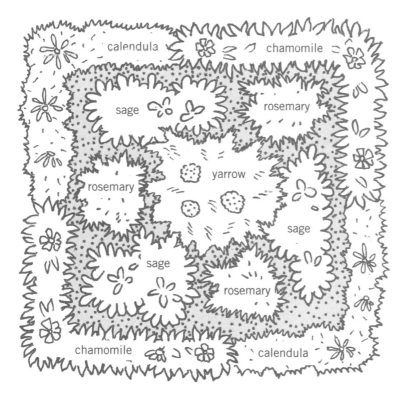

Plot Garden Plants

- 3 sage
- 3 rosemary
- 2 yarrow
- 21 chamomile
- 21 calendula

HAIR CARE RECIPES

Simple and effective are two words you could use to describe these recipes, because hair care should involve minimal fuss.

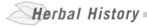

Use this herbal vinegar diluted with equal amounts of water to give your hair shine. Traditionally, sage and rosemary were used for dark hair; yarrow, chamomile, and calendula for light hair. Rinsing with an infusion of these herbs won't change your hair color, however, unless you do so while catching the liquid in a basin to pour over your hair repeatedly for several weeks. Even then the change will be quite subtle. (Before using, test for skin sensitivity using the patch test; see page 10.)

> Equal amounts fresh herbs of your choice from the Hair Care Garden
> Cider vinegar

Fill a clean jar with one dried or fresh herb of your choice. Cover with cider vinegar and place in a sunny window. After about 2 weeks, strain the herbs from the vinegar. Use equal parts of this rinse and water on your hair after shampooing.

This herbal vinegar may also be used diluted to half strength with water to use as a skin toner. (See the Skin Care Garden on page 136.)

Herbal History

- When planted with rue, sage was said to keep toads away.
- A conserve, or jamlike preparation, of sage flowers was said to aid the brain and nervous system.
- Legend has it that rosemary's flowers are blue because the Virgin Mary draped her blue cloak over a rosemary bush, causing the flowers to turn that color.

Fragrant Hair Rinse

Massage this rinse into your hair after shampooing, then dry and style your hair as usual. Make up your rinse the night before you use it and store it in the refrigerator.

1 quart water
1 cup fresh or ½ cup dried rosemary

Heat the water to boiling in an enamel or stainless-steel saucepan. Add the rosemary. Remove the mixture from the heat, cover, and let steep for 15 minutes. Strain the herb and store the herb-infused water in a glass jar in the refrigerator. Use within 48 hours.

READING LABELS

Herbal hair-care products are currently a popular trend. By reading the labels, you can see what the ingredients really are. You might be surprised to find that there are little herb-derived ingredients in them.

Ingredients on product labels are listed in order from the largest amount to the smallest amount included in the product. After looking at some of these products, I think you will find that the products contain more herbs when you make them yourself. (For information on books that have more herbal hair-care recipes, see Recommended Reading.)

Headache Relief Garden

This is a lush and colorful bed of herbs to enjoy visually. Working in this garden will be an aromatic pleasure as well, and if the stress of the day has started to take its toll on you in the form of a tension headache, sit and relax in or near the garden for a while, picking some sprigs of herb to enjoy. This will help you to divert your thoughts from any worries that you might have.

PLOT GARDEN

Arrange the plants so that the lemon balm is centrally located in the bed. Plant the feverfew next to it on one side, and the chamomile plants on the other side. Arrange the plantings of lavender in a curve to the side and front of the feverfew. The lavender's flowers look pretty with those of the feverfew.

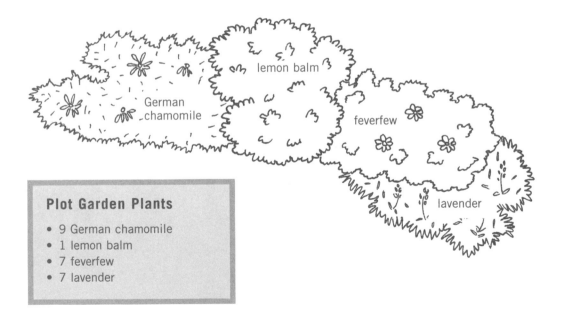

Plot Garden Plants

- 9 German chamomile
- 1 lemon balm
- 7 feverfew
- 7 lavender

lavender

lemon balm

feverfew

German chamomile

CONTAINER GARDEN

For a container variation, plant the herbs from this garden in cedar boxes 2 feet long by 1 foot wide and however tall you want them to be. You can vary the height of each container for interest. If you are feeling ambitious and crafty, you can make containers of varying heights. Troughs of different sizes, materials, and designs are available commercially. Do not use treated wood for this container project or any other gardening project; the chemicals used in the treatment of the wood can leach into the soil and subsequently into the plants.

Each individual herb is planted in its own box. Arrange the boxes so that a right angle is formed. A small piece of garden statuary would look good in this corner. The tallest box may be placed in the corner or on one end. It is a flexible design; the box heights may be staggered from tallest to shortest if you choose, or even at random heights.

To make a unique and interesting planter that is quite portable, take an old chair that has a worn-out cane seat and tack a piece of canvas securely to the seat frame, letting the canvas sag down several inches to form a container. Line the canvas section with black plastic that has a few holes punched in it. Fill with potting mix and plant herbs in it.

Another idea is to arrange containers of herbs on the sides of steps (make sure there is enough room for people to manage the steps safely). You can also place containers of plants on various rungs of a stepladder. Balance wide boards on the rungs on either side of the ladder; be sure the boards are level. Place containers of plants on them.

Container Garden Plants

- 3 lavender
- 2 lemon balm
- 5 feverfew
- 7 German chamomile

HEADACHE RELIEF RECIPES

Most of us lead busy lives that are full of distractions and a variety of stresses. Take pause and allow some simple herb preparations to aid you in relieving the headaches associated with such lifestyles.

Headache Relief Tea

This tea can help you to relax, and relieves headaches that are caused by tension.

> 1 teaspoon dried or 2 teaspoons fresh lemon balm or chamomile blossoms
> 1 cup boiling water

Place the fresh or dried lemon balm or chamomile blossoms in the boiling water. Cover and infuse for 15 minutes, then strain. Sip slowly.

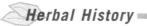

Herbal History

- Lemon balm was mixed with honey and smeared inside beehives to attract new swarms of bees.
- Crushed lemon-balm leaves were applied to rabid dog bites.
- Along with other herbs, many Shaker communities planted and raised feverfew in their gardens.

Headache Band

I'm sure many of you have seen these available in stores. They are simple to make and much more economical, too!

Dried lavender buds
1 12-inch long by 3-inch wide fabric pouch

Distribute the dried lavender buds evenly throughout the fabric pouch. Stitch through the pouch at 2-inch intervals. Place on your forehead and over closed eyes when you have a headache. Rest and enjoy the aroma.

Healthy Heart Garden

$\mathcal{G}$rowing cayenne peppers and garlic and using them in your diet will help maintain a healthy cardiovascular system. Both of these plants are usually grown in vegetable gardens, but, by moving them into your herb gardens you will be giving them a unique and easily accessible home.

CONTAINER GARDEN

Garlic and cayenne pepper plants can easily be container-grown; just remember that they need full sun and good drainage. Plant three garlic cloves in a 12-inch-wide container, and one clove in a shorter container that is 8 inches wide. Plant cayenne in a 10-inch-wide container that is in between the heights of the other two containers. After the plants are established, mulch the surface of the potting mix or cover the surface lightly with smooth pebbles for interest.

Alternately, you can plant the garlic and cayenne separately in square planters near your kitchen door for easy access to the herbal harvest.

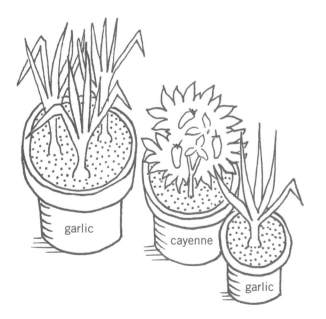

garlic

cayenne

garlic

Container Garden Plants
• 4 garlic cloves
• 1 cayenne

PLOT GARDEN

Although they're not commonly thought of as decorative plants, garlic's spikes of foliage and cayenne pepper's red fruits can make a lovely show in an herb bed. These herbs can also easily be incorporated into your vegetable garden. Remember that if your climate experiences hard freezes, you should plant the garlic cloves in fall and mulch after the ground has frozen hard. The mulch keeps the ground from heaving and "ejecting" the cloves. This garden will do best if grown in a fully sunny spot.

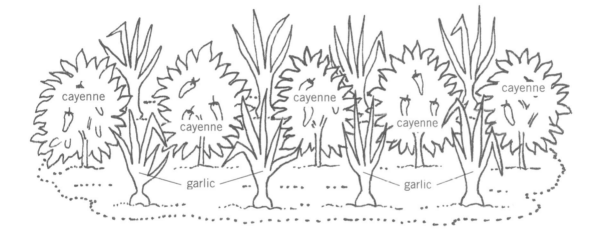

NATURAL FOOD STORE NOTES

As the owner and proprietor of Franklin Cornucopia, Nancy Kirklin meets a lot of customers seeking herbs to treat their ills. Some of her customers find parsley tea to be a nutrition-booster. They buy cayenne to improve circulation and immune-system function, and garlic for lowering blood pressure.

HEALTHY HEART RECIPES

Having fresh herbal harvests will give you the pleasure of well-seasoned foods. Try these recipes, and open up your cookbooks to explore additional ideas.

Cayenne Garlic Seasoning

This is a versatile recipe that adds lots of flavor to a variety of foods. Use it while your harvest is fresh, and freeze some for winter use.

2 bulbs of garlic, cloves separated and peeled
1 cayenne pepper, stem and seeds removed (use gloves!)
Vinegar (rice or white-wine vinegar is good)

Place the garlic cloves and pepper in your food processor and finely chop them. Place tablespoon-size portions on a cookie sheet and freeze, then transfer to a freezer bag for storage. Do not add any vinegar to a mixture intended for freezing.

An alternate way to store this seasoning is to place the chopped mixture in a jar and pour vinegar over it to cover. Store in the refrigerator. Use the mixture a tablespoon at a time in soups, stir-fries, dips, and whatever else suits your fancy. The infused vinegar can be used separately as a hot and flavorful addition to salad dressings and soups, or as a meat marinade.

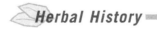 **Herbal History**

- Hot peppers were said to grow better if planted by a hot-tempered person.
- Garlic is also known as the "stinking rose."

Salsa

Low-fat and packed with flavor and nutrients, this recipe can serve many purposes.

- 5 large tomatoes, peeled, cored, seeded, and chopped
- 1 large onion, peeled and chopped
- 1–3 cayenne peppers, seeded and chopped (use 3 peppers if you like your salsa to have a lot of heat)
- 2 cloves garlic, peeled and chopped
- Salt to taste (no more than ½ teaspoon)
- 1 tablespoon chopped fresh cilantro (if available)

Combine all ingredients. Can be used as a dip, topping, or as an ingredient in various recipes.

Garlic Spread

This recipe is good on raw veggies or as a condiment for sandwiches.

- 1 cup mayonnaise (you may use fat-free, if desired)
- 6 cloves garlic, peeled
- 2 tablespoons lemon juice
- ¼ teaspoon freshly ground black pepper
- Pinch salt

Place the mayonnaise, garlic, and lemon juice in a food processor and blend well. Add the salt and pepper. Refrigerate until ready to serve.

Mouth Care Garden

Many herbs are useful for mouth care, which comes as a surprise to a lot of people when they hear it. Once again, nature's bounty proves its worth in a unique way. The following garden plans will help you get started.

CONTAINER GARDEN

Place this garden's plants in a large container for an interesting variation. Buy an inexpensive plastic kiddy pool and punch a lot of holes in the bottom for drainage. Place the container in its permanent spot (when it is full, it will be heavy and difficult to move). Fill with a light potting mix to facilitate drainage.

Plant the dill or fennel plants in the center. Around the inside perimeter of the pool, alternate plantings of parsley, thyme, and sage. Stack stones or bricks around the plastic pool to cover it and add decorative interest; tuck some low-growing thyme plants such as mother of thyme, red creeping thyme, or white creeping thyme into the cracks between the stones. As they grow, they will soften the lines of the stones.

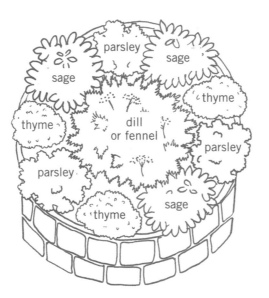

Container Garden Plants

- 2 dill or fennel
- 3 parsley
- 3 thyme
- 3 sage

PLOT GARDEN

A kidney-shaped bed will nicely hold the herbs in this garden. The dill or fennel plants will bloom the first year; the parsley will bloom the second year, since it is a biennial. Italian and curly parsley can be used interchangeably. Use the low-growing thyme to fill in the empty spaces.

The umbel flowers of some of the plants in this garden are attractive to butterflies and other beneficial insects that aid in garden pest control. The parsley, dill, and fennel plants sometimes attract the caterpillars of the swallowtail butterfly; if you find that they're eating all of your parsley, cut some sprigs off your existing plants or buy some cut parsley at the grocery store. Leave this on the ground and relocate the caterpillars from your plants.

Plot Garden Plants

- 3 dill or fennel
- 3 sage
- 3 parsley
- 4 low-growing thyme

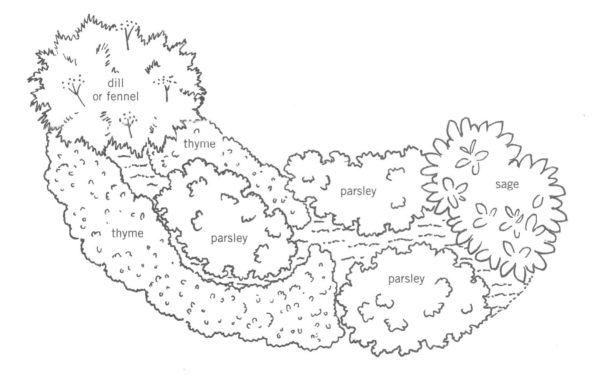

MOUTH CARE RECIPES

These recipes echo the way herbs were used in the times prior to commercial mouth-care preparations. They are quite simple to make and economical, too.

Sage Tooth Scrub

Sage's ability to inhibit bacterial growth makes it a good ingredient for a tooth cleaner.

    1   teaspoon dried sage leaf
    1   teaspoon salt

Grind the sage in a food processor or coffee grinder. Add the salt and mix. Sprinkle a small amount of the mixture on a dampened toothbrush. Brush your teeth as usual.

NATURAL BREATH FRESHENER

Sometimes, between tooth brushings, we could use an extra breath freshener. The answer might just be sitting on your lunch plate. After eating, thoroughly chew and swallow a sprig of parsley. The naturally ocurring chlorophyll in the parsley acts as an odor neutralizer, and you'll get the added benefit of vitamins and minerals.

As an alternative, try thoroughly chewing and swallowing a teaspoon of dried dill or fennel seeds. These two herbs are more strongly flavored than the parsley, but work just as well.

Antiseptic Mouth Rinse

Thyme's antibacterial properties make this rinse appropriate for daily use as a deodorizing mouth rinse or for occasional use when you have a canker sore. Any leftovers can be refrigerated, but must be used the next day.

1 teaspoon dried or 2 teaspoons fresh thyme
1 cup boiling water

Add the thyme to the boiling water. Cover and steep for 15 minutes. Strain, and let cool to lukewarm. Use as a gargle.

Herbal History

- Gardeners throughout time have considered it unlucky to move parsley from an old house to a new one.
- In Old World Germany, brides carried bouquets of dill.
- It is said that if you wipe your eyes with a sprig of thyme, you can see fairies.

Rejuvenation Garden

*T*he word "rejuvenate" means to restore, to stimulate, to renew. The plants included in this garden are meant to aid you in all of these things. The unique plant combinations will make visitors to your garden take notice, and the herbs will provide you with an interesting visual display, as well.

PLOT GARDEN

An oval-shaped bed is an interesting way to display the herbs in this garden. Identical plantings mirror each other on both sides of the bed. Lay black plastic covered with gravel or stones between plantings. Curly parsley makes a more attractive display than Italian parsley.

Plant your herb garden next to and hanging from the porch for easy harvest and ready enjoyment. Or, you could plant this garden along the wall of your house, placing a garden plaque of an appropriate design on the wall for decoration and to keep watch over your herbs.

Plot Garden Plants

- 3 red clover
- 2 cayenne
- 8 garlic cloves
- 6 parsley

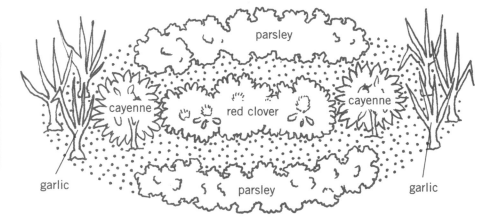

CONTAINER GARDEN

To keep hanging baskets from drying out so quickly, particularly the wire models that are lined with coconut fiber, line them with a plastic bag in which you've punched a few holes, then add potting mix. Plant each basket with 1 red clover and 1 parsley plant. Plant the cayenne and garlic cloves in the ground along the edge of the porch or in a long trough container.

Container Garden Plants

- 2 red clover
- 2 parsley
- 2 cayenne
- 5 garlic cloves

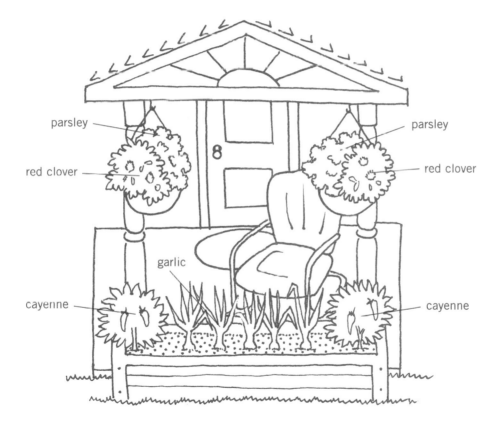

parsley

red clover

parsley

red clover

garlic

cayenne

cayenne

REJUVENATION RECIPES

Healthful fare that liberally uses herbs will go a long way in your well-being. Take advantage of these herbs while they are fresh — they are a pleasing addition to your table.

Fresh Garden Vegetables

This recipe is packed with vitamins and minerals. It provides your table with a lot of color and flavor. Use whatever vegetables happen to be ripe in your garden.

  1 tablespoon olive oil
  3 garlic cloves, peeled and chopped
Approximately 3 cups assorted coarsely chopped vegetables
     from your garden
½ teaspoon dried cayenne, ground
½ cup chopped parsley
Dash of salt
½–1 cup red clover sprouts (see page 159)

1. In a large skillet, heat the olive oil. Add the chopped garlic and sauté over high heat until it changes color. Add the chopped vegetables and sauté on medium-high heat until they are crisp but tender. This will take 10 to 20 minutes depending on the vegetables you are including. Remove the skillet from the heat.
2. Add the cayenne, parsley, and salt, and mix well. Before serving, sprinkle the vegetables with red clover sprouts.

Herbal History

- Garlic is supposed to have been introduced to Europe by the crusaders.
- Folklore holds that parsley seeds must go to the devil and return nine times before they sprout!
- In times before refrigeration, liberal use of herbs helped mask the taste and smell of spoiled food.

Rejuvenation Tea

Stop what you're doing and sip some of this tea. It will help you get back on track.

    1   cup boiling water
    2   teaspoons fresh clover blossoms
    2   teaspoons fresh parsley leaves, chopped
  ¼–1   teaspoon honey

Pour water over the herbs. Cover, and steep for 15 minutes. Strain the herbs, and add honey. Sip slowly.

Pita Dip

The spicy ingredients make this a great party appetizer.

½ cup sesame tahini	¼ teaspoon dried cayenne, ground
½ cup water	¼ teaspoon salt
1 tablespoon lemon juice	2 tablespoons fresh parsley, chopped
4 garlic cloves, peeled and finely chopped	3 pita rounds, cut into 2-inch wedges

Mix all ingredients except parsley and pita wedges. Place the mixture in a serving bowl and sprinkle with parsley. Arrange pita wedges around the bowl, and serve.

HOW TO REJUVENATE

It all sounds so easy. Eat right, exercise, and reduce stress, and you will feel better physically. The stressors that keep us off balance mentally and physically often can be hard to deal with. Take a hard look at your lifestyle and habits. Then, use some herbs to help support your efforts at changing your lifestyle into a healthier one.

Take 5 minutes each day in a quiet place for serious relaxation. For example, sit comfortably, close your eyes, and take some deep breaths.

Add some form of exercise to your daily activities. Start with 10–15 minutes a day and work yourself up gradually.

Make one healthy change in your diet per week.

Relaxation Garden

This garden will be attractive to pollinators such as honeybees, so plant it near your vegetable garden, fruit trees, or any other plants in need of pollination. The variety of blooms, scents, and foliage in this garden is both interesting and beautiful. All of these herbs have a reputation for calming the nerves and promoting relaxation. Read the individual herb profiles for each plant to determine which ones are best suited for you.

CONTAINER GARDEN

To grow this garden in containers, first plant valerian in the ground at the center of the garden (it is too tall to plant in a container). Surround it with four troughs that contain separate plantings of the four other plants.

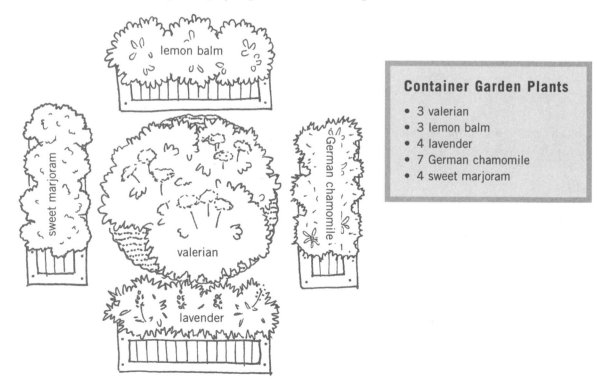

Container Garden Plants

- 3 valerian
- 3 lemon balm
- 4 lavender
- 7 German chamomile
- 4 sweet marjoram

PLOT GARDEN

This garden would look attractive planted against a fence. Valerian is the tallest and should be planted at the back of your Relaxation Garden. Plant lavender directly in front of the valerian, with lemon balm and German chamomile on either side of the lavender. Plant sweet marjoram in front of the lavender. The aromas of the flowers and/or foliage of these plants is relaxation therapy on its own.

For a charming variation, try making an herb "bed." Use sections of picket fencing of two different heights for the head and foot of the bed, and plant the herbs inside. If you find the headboard and footboard of an old bed at a garage sale, they, too, can be used at either end of the herb planting.

> ### Plot Garden Plants
>
> - 3 valerian
> - 2 lemon balm
> - 8 German chamomile
> - 5 lavender
> - 3 sweet marjoram

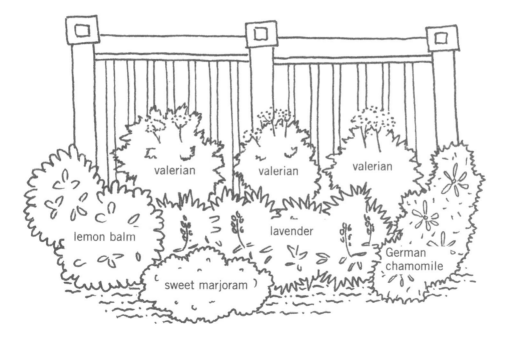

RELAXATION RECIPES

Using these recipes to promote relaxation provides you with an excuse to halt the pace of your life, if only for a few minutes. Stop and sit to sip a cup of Relaxing Tea, or rest for a few moments while sniffing a Relaxation Inhaler. Just taking a moment of time out of your busy day will help a lot toward giving your body and mind a rest.

Relaxing Tea

Sipping a cup of aromatic tea will give you a few moments of quiet time.

1   teaspoon dried lemon balm or dried chamomile blossoms
1   cup boiling water

Add the lemon balm or chamomile blossoms to the boiling water. Cover and infuse for 15 minutes. Strain the herbs from the infusion and sip slowly.

NATURAL FOOD STORE NOTES

The customers of Nature's Cupboard in Greenwood, Indiana, find valerian to be a sleep aid. They also use it as a muscle relaxer. Due to valerian's unpleasant smell and taste, most people prefer to take valerian in capsule form rather than as a tincture.

Relaxation Inhaler

This little bag of herbs can be kept on your desk at work, on the dashboard of your car, on a windowsill at home, or anywhere that you might want a quick de-stressor. How relaxing the scents are!

1 tablespoon dried lavender buds
1 tablespoon dried marjoram
1 tablespoon dried lemon balm
1 tablespoon dried chamomile
1 muslin tea bag

Add all of the dried herbs to the muslin bag, and close the bag snugly. When the herbs lose their aroma, empty the contents of the bag into the compost and replace with more dried herbs.

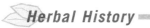

Herbal History

- For a time, valerian root was used to scent linen.
- Lemon balm was only used as an attractant to bees for the first thousand years that it was cultivated.
- Essential oil of lavender was popularly used to prevent swooning or fainting.

Skin Care Garden

*T*hese herbs can be planted to enjoy for their flowers' colors and good aromas. The use of the harvested herbs is equally enjoyable to help you care for your skin naturally. Each herb can be used for different skin types and conditions. (See page 139.)

CONTAINER GARDEN

A half whiskey barrel is a perfect-sized container for the herbal skin-care garden. When it's full of potting mix, a whiskey barrel is heavy, so place it where you want to keep it before you fill. Plant the lavender, German chamomile, and calendula, then place the prostrate rosemary so that its foliage tumbles over the edge of the container.

Another interesting option is to place an old metal tub or basin on its side with about a third of it buried in the ground. Plant the herbs so that they appear to be spilling out of the tub.

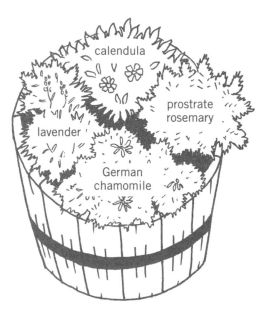

Container Garden Plants

- 2 lavender
- 5 German chamomile
- 5 calendula
- 1 prostrate rosemary

PLOT GARDEN

The height and size of the plants in this garden make it perfect to serve as a classic sundial herb planting. The herbs' flowers will add color. A birdbath or gazing ball could be used in place of the sundial; in the latter case, the purple, blue, bright yellow or orange, and yellow and white blooms of each respective herb would be reflected off the gazing ball's shiny surface. Place crushed brick or stone around the perimeter of the garden and between the four different plantings to divide them.

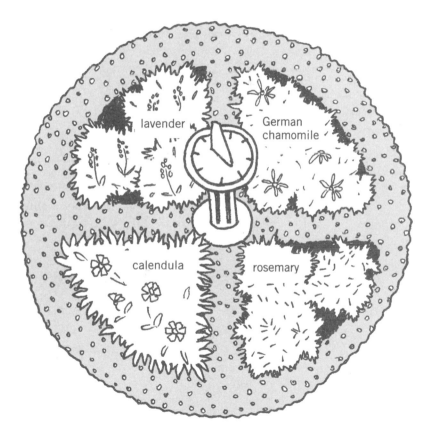

Plot Garden Plants

- 3 lavender
- 3 rosemary
- 5 calendula
- 5 German chamomile

SKIN CARE RECIPES

Herbs combined with other natural ingredients will go a long way toward keeping your skin in good condition.

Multipurpose Skin Solution

You may be surprised to see an herbal vinegar listed in the skin-care section of this book, but herbal vinegars indeed are a good way to transfer the benefits of the herbs into a liquid form that can benefit the skin.

Rosemary is good for oily skin and is also deodorizing. Lavender is appropriate for any skin type. Calendula's antibacterial properties make it good for blemished skin. Chamomile can be helpful to sensitive skin, and its toning qualities make it a great aftershave soother for men. Before using, try a small amount of the substance on your skin in a patch test. (See page 10.)

½–1 cup dried or fresh Skin Care Garden herb of your choice
   2 cups cider vinegar
Distilled water

1. Add the herbs to the cider vinegar in a noncorrosive pan and simmer, covered, for 30 minutes. Remove from the heat and allow to cool.
2. Strain the herbs from the vinegar, squeezing to get as much vinegar from them as possible. Dilute this vinegar with an equal amount of distilled water and use as a facial toner or after-bath skin splash.

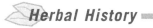

Herbal History

- Calendula was used by the cultures of India and Arabia prior to its introduction to ancient Greece.
- Some gardeners believe that if chamomile is planted next to a sick or dying plant, it will be revived.
- People have slept with rosemary leaves placed under their pillows to prevent nightmares.

Gentle Skin Scrub

This scrub is gentle enough for facial care but is also effective on other parts of your body. To avoid making a mess on your bathroom floor, stand in the tub or shower when rubbing it on your body. The scrub will stimulate your skin while removing dead skin cells. The mixture will keep indefinitely as long as it doesn't get wet.

    1   tablespoon dried lavender buds, finely ground
    1   tablespoon dried rosemary, finely ground
    ½   cup oatmeal, coarsely ground

Combine the herbs and oatmeal; store in a covered glass jar. To use, place a teaspoonful of the mixture in your hand, moisten with a little water, and rub gently on your skin in a circular motion. Rinse the residue off and towel dry.

Calendula Skin Soother

Use this infused oil to soothe irritated skin.

For calendula-infused oil, fill a very clean jar that has a tight-fitting lid with dried calendula blossoms. Cover the blossoms with olive oil. Place in a sunny windowsill for 2 weeks.

Strain out the blossoms, reserving the oil. Refill the jar with more dried calendula blossoms. Pour in the reserved oil, and add more if needed to cover the herbs. Place jar in a paper bag and let sit in a sunny windowsill for 2 more weeks.

Strain and store in a dark glass bottle. Add 800 IU vitamin E to the oil to enhance its keeping qualities. Store in a dark, cool place.

Herbal Salve

Calendula salve is what my son carries in his first-aid kit when he is camping. It's terrific for rashes, minor cuts, scrapes, and insect bites.

    4½ tablespoons calendula-infused oil (see also page 12)
    2   tablespoons grated beeswax
    2   400 IU vitamin E capsules

Melt oil and beeswax in a heatproof container over boiling water. Remove from the heat and add contents of vitamin E capsules. Store in a low, widemouthed jar.

WHICH HERB TO CHOOSE?

Each of the herbs planted in the Skin Care Garden offers you unique skin-conditioning qualities.

Lavender is appropriate for all skin types. It is deodorizing and cleansing. Lavender can also be used to help relieve mild sunburn discomfort. Use the flower buds.

Calendula is effective on skin suffering from rashes and acne. Also good for oily skin, calendula's antibacterial properties make it helpful in healing blemishes. Use the flower petals.

Chamomile is good for sensitive skin, and it has a gentle effect on dry skin. Use the flowers.

Rosemary is best used on oily skin. It has astringent properties, is deodorizing, refreshing, and stimulating. Use the leaves.

Sore Muscle Care Garden

The herbs included in this garden will do well in a warm, dappled-sunlight situation. In North America the best way to raise ginger is in a container, so it can be moved inside when cold weather hits. I also like growing rosemary in containers, rather than digging it up to move inside for cold weather, because the plants usually don't like being uprooted.

PLOT GARDEN

Plant ginger in one container and rosemary in another. Plant the sweet marjoram around the bases of the two containers. Keep in mind that the ginger will require more water than the rosemary or sweet marjoram.

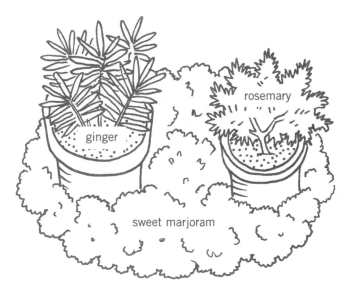

ginger

rosemary

sweet marjoram

> **Plot Garden Plants**
>
> - 1 ginger rhizome
> - 1 rosemary
> - 5 sweet marjoram

CONTAINER GARDEN

For a staggered container planting, place one rosemary plant in a round container taller than the others, one ginger rhizome in a square, medium-height container, and three sweet marjoram plants in a low, circular container. The different heights and shapes of the containers will add interest to the plantings. Elevate the containers on a table or stand: If you have sore muscles, you won't want to be bending over containers on the ground!

For a rustic look, line a wooden box or crate with black plastic, poking holes in the bottom for drainage. Fill with potting mix and plant the herbs in it.

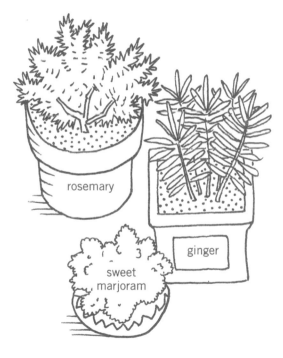

rosemary

ginger

sweet marjoram

Container Garden Plants

- 1 rosemary
- 1 ginger rhizome
- 3 sweet marjoram

SORE MUSCLE RECIPES

When you have sore muscles from overwork or mild strains, these recipes should help you to obtain relief. For severe sprains, strains, and muscle soreness, seek the care of a health-care professional.

Herb Infused Muscle Rub

Sweet marjoram or rosemary can be made into an infused massage oil.

Equal parts dried herbs and olive oil

Follow any one of the three recipes for making herbal infused oil on pages 12–13.

Massage the oil into sore, overworked muscles.

Store the remaining oil in a dark glass bottle that is labeled with its contents. Keep the bottle in a cool dark place.

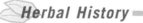

Herbal History

- Jamaica's ginger has long been considered the best in the world.
- Germans call sweet marjoram wurstkraut, or "sausage herb."
- Rosemary was burned by monks for fumigation purposes.

Sore Foot Soak

Add this bath bag to a basin of very warm water and soak the soreness of your feet away. You might want to place a towel on the floor under the basin to catch any spills.

About ¼ cup grated fresh ginger
1 muslin bath bag

Place the grated ginger in a muslin bath bag. Let the bag steep in a basin of very warm water for 15 minutes, then place your feet in the water. Soak your feet for 30 minutes, then towel dry.

Sore Muscle Wrap

The warmth of towels soaked in an herbal infusion will help relieve minor muscle soreness. The infusion should be warm, not hot; after removal, the skin will appear pink or reddened. Too high a temperature will cause skin burns. Be sure to do a patch test (see page 10) before using, and do not use this treatment more than once a day.

2 quarts water
2 cups fresh or 1 cup dried rosemary leaves or sweet marjoram leaves

Heat water in a saucepan until simmering. Add herbs and simmer, covered, for 10 minutes. Strain the infusion into a basin or large bowl. Allow to cool slightly. Soak an old towel or piece of flannel in the herbal infusion; wring out until just moist. Apply the cloth to the sore area, and rest the wrapped area on a covered surface. Keep the wrap in place for 15 minutes.

NATURAL FOOD STORE NOTES

Customers at Franklin Cornucopia use rosemary to improve both circulation and liver function. However, they are cautious when taking rosemary internally — overuse can be toxic.

Throat Care Garden

This group of herbs is practically carefree after they are planted. All three are drought-tolerant and resistant to insects. Don't overlook the wonderful culinary uses of each of these plants; fitting to herbs' reputations as multiuse plants, any of these three herbs will season a variety of dishes.

CONTAINER GARDEN

A simple trough garden is an appropriate alternative for these plants. If you wish, nestle a small piece of statuary or a whimsical garden stake among them.

For a more elaborate display, plant individual herbs in separate containers of different sizes and shapes, and arrange them according to the space you have available.

Container Garden Plants

- 1 thyme
- 1 sage
- 1 sweet marjoram

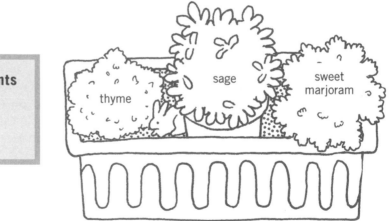

PLOT GARDEN

The low-growing habit of the herbs in this garden make it a good choice for a rock garden. To obtain rocks of the size and shape that you want, ask around at excavation and roadwork sites. Usually the workers will be happy to give you some. Just be sure to ask permission first, and choose rocks that you can manage to transport to your garden. Around your plants, arrange as many rocks as you need to create a pleasing appearance. You can also sink concrete blocks sideways into the ground, planting the herbs in their openings.

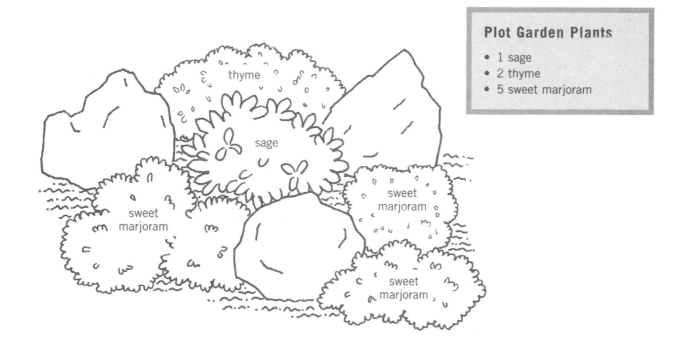

Plot Garden Plants

- 1 sage
- 2 thyme
- 5 sweet marjoram

THROAT CARE RECIPES

The following recipes offer you simple and quick ways to treat a mild sore throat. In addition to these treatments, get plenty of rest.

Helpful Throat Gargle

This infusion also can be sipped warm with a little honey added to aid in soothing a sore throat and/or raspy voice.

- 1 teaspoon dried or 2 teaspoons fresh Throat Care Garden herb of your choice
- 1 cup boiling water

Add the herbs in the boiling water, cover, and infuse for 10 to 15 minutes. Let cool to lukewarm and use for a gargle. Do not swallow. Leftover infusion may be refrigerated for use within 48 hours.

Herbal Sore Throat Relief Broth

This is a warming drink to soothe a scratchy throat, but drink no more than one to two cups per day.

- ½ teaspoon dried or 1 teaspoon fresh sage
- ½ teaspoon dried or 1 teaspoon fresh sweet marjoram
- 1 cup boiling water
- Pinch of salt

Place the herbs in a heatproof cup or mug. Pour the boiling water over the herbs. Cover and let steep 10 minutes, then strain out the herbs. Stir in salt. Sip slowly.

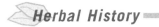

Herbal History

- Aphrodite, the Greek goddess of love, was said to have created sweet marjoram.
- The antiseptic properties of thyme's essential oil were discovered in 1725 by a German apothecary.

Healing Herbal Vapors

Reminiscent of the vaporizing treatments many of us received as children, this treatment can aid in soothing irritated throats. Use caution with hot steam; it can burn the skin if you are too close for a long period of time.

- 1 quart boiling water
- ¼ cup dried or ½ cup fresh thyme
- ¼ cup dried or ½ cup fresh sweet marjoram

Place the herbs in a large metal or glass bowl on a table that you can easily lean over. Pour the boiling water over the herbs. Lean over the bowl and, without getting too close, inhale the steam. Breathe deeply until the steam feels too hot on your face, then remove your face from the steam. Continue this pattern for 15 to 20 minutes, or until the mixture cools.

Singer's Tea

Marjoram tea is a traditional remedy that singers use to combat hoarseness. If the only singing you do is in the shower, sip this tea when you are suffering from a scratchy throat or raspy voice. Without the honey, this recipe can be used as a gargle.

- 1 tablespoon fresh or 2 teaspoons dried marjoram leaves
- 1 teaspoon fresh or ½ teaspoon dried thyme leaves
- 1 cup boiling water
- 1 teaspoon honey

Pour boiling water over the herbs; cover and let steep 10 minutes. Strain, and add honey. Sip slowly. When using this tea as a gargle, omit the honey and allow the infusion to cool to lukewarm before gargling.

Traveler's Herb Garden

*I*n my opinion, these herbs are essential to have along while traveling. No one expects illness or injury when away from home, but it doesn't hurt to be prepared for minor emergencies.

CONTAINER GARDEN

For a variation on this garden, plant the ginger and aloe in different-sized pots. Place them next to each other in front of echinacea planted in the ground. Plant the German chamomile in the ground in front of the two containers.

Alternately, you could arrange the separate containers of herbs in a plastic-lined basket; tuck Spanish moss around them to stabilize, anchor, and conceal the containers. Another idea is to line a large old basket (such as a wicker laundry basket) with black plastic, punching holes in the bottom for drainage. Add moistened potting mix and plants.

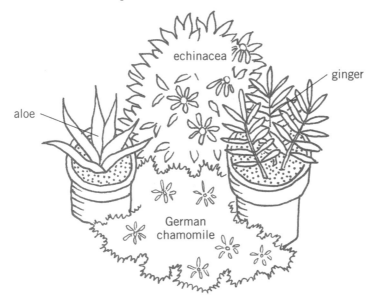

Container Garden Plants

- 3 echinacea
- 9 German chamomile
- 1 aloe
- 1 ginger rhizome

PLOT GARDEN

Plant the aloe and ginger in layered dishes, with the ginger on the bottom dish; keep the soil in this bottom dish very moist. Place smooth stones on the surface of the soil around the aloe and ginger plantings. Plant the echinacea behind the two containers. Arrange the two containers with one on top of the other. Plant the German chamomile in the left front side of the containers.

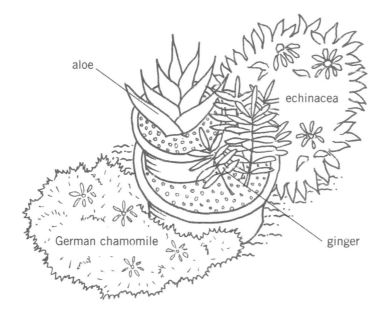

aloe

echinacea

German chamomile

ginger

Plot Garden Plants

- 3 echinacea
- 5 German chamomile
- 1 aloe
- 1 ginger rhizome

TRAVELER'S RECIPES

Pack all of your herbal travel kit carefully to avoid breakage. Plastic bubble wrap is very helpful protection for containers. For international travel, stick to commercial products with clear labels to avoid problems when going through customs.

Travel Kit

To assure trouble-free traveling, pack the following herbs "just in case."

1 small bottle commercial aloe vera gel (4–8 ounces)
1 bottle (about ½ cup) candied gingerroot (see the recipe on page 95)
1 bottle echinacea root, ground up and placed in capsules (20 capsules), or
    1 bottle (about 1 ounce) echinacea-root tincture (see page 13)
1 small package (1 cup) dried chamomile blossoms
1 muslin tea bag
Several adhesive bandages

Use the aloe gel for: minor sunburns, cuts, scrapes, or insect bites.
Use the candied gingerroot for: any gastrointestinal upset or travel sickness.
Use the echinacea root capsules or tincture for: immune system boosting at the first sign of illness.
Use the chamomile for: minor stomach upsets, promotion of relaxation and/or sleep. You can also make a chamomile infusion and soak a clean cloth with it, placing it over tired and irritated eyes. The infusion can be added to your bathwater for an herbal bath.

Chamomile Dream Pillow

Make this small pillow ahead of time and take it with you when traveling. The fruity, applelike aroma will help you relax, making for easier sleep — even in a strange place.

2 6-inch squares of tightly woven fabric, or 2 washcloths
2 cups dried chamomile flowers

With right sides together, sew up 3 sides of the fabric squares. Turn right side out, and fill the pouch loosely with chamomile flowers. Sew closed the open end. Insert dream pillow between your pillow and pillow case before going to sleep.

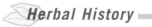

Herbal History

- Echinacea is a Greek word meaning "hedge hog."
- Some Native American women used echinacea's dried flower heads as combs.
- Chamomile has been planted in garden seats so that when you sit down, the herb's fragrance is released.

Tummy Care Garden

A variety of herbs are included in the Tummy Care Garden. It is nice to know that there are so many plants that can help to remedy an upset stomach. This garden will attract honeybees to help with the pollination of plants in other parts of your garden. Also, beneficial insects are attracted to the umbel flowers of the fennel and dill plants.

CONTAINER GARDEN

An interesting variation on this garden uses stacked containers of gradually reduced sizes placed one atop the other; this makes a beautiful presentation. Set these plantings up where you will want to keep them, because they will be too heavy to move after you have filled the containers.

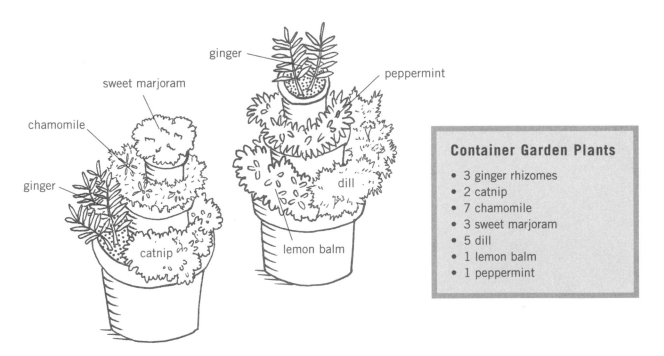

Container Garden Plants

- 3 ginger rhizomes
- 2 catnip
- 7 chamomile
- 3 sweet marjoram
- 5 dill
- 1 lemon balm
- 1 peppermint

PLOT GARDEN

This plan will make a large bed in which you could place a bench to sit and enjoy the plants surrounding you. Place mulch near the front of the bed, and the bench nearby. For easier maintenance, put black plastic down before laying the mulch to help keep weeds from growing up through it. Place the fennel or dill in the back left corner of the bed. Plant lemon balm next to it, and catnip to the right of the lemon balm. Peppermint should be planted in a container and then sunk in the ground in the back right corner. Plant the chamomile in front of the peppermint, bringing the chamomile planting out toward the front of the bed. Plant the sweet marjoram in front of the fennel or dill, lemon balm, and catnip. The ginger rhizome should be planted in a container and placed on the left-hand side of the bed.

For a different arrangement, plant groups of these herbs along a path to make an herb walk. Add a pottery plant marker next to each group to identify the herbs.

> **Plot Garden Plants**
>
> - 3 fennel or 5 dill
> - 2 lemon balm
> - 2 catnip
> - 1 peppermint
> - 9 German chamomile
> - 7 sweet marjoram
> - 1 ginger rhizome

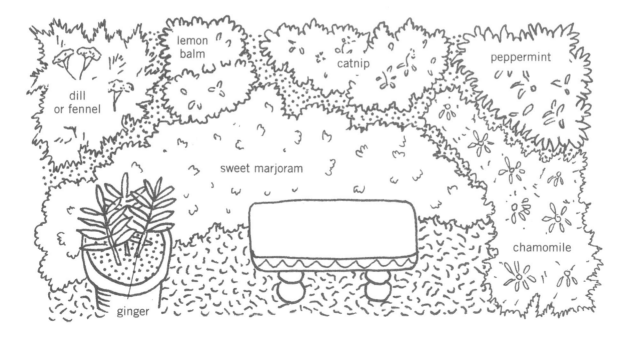

TUMMY CARE RECIPES

Many quick-fix medicines for stomach upset are advertised on television every day. Save some money and try these herbal remedies instead.

Tummy Tea

The herbal mix of this tea makes it effective for treating stomach upsets resulting from too much food, acid indigestion, or mild stomach cramping. Make this tea ahead of time by placing 2 teaspoons of the herbal mix in heat-sealable tea bags, seal, and store in a glass container. Then your tea is available in an easy-to-use form when needed.

> Equal parts dried catnip, dried lemon balm, dried peppermint, and dried sweet marjoram
> 1 cup boiling water

Mix the herbs. Add 2 teaspoons of this mix to the boiling water and infuse for 15 minutes. Strain and sip slowly. Store the remaining dried herbs in a glass container away from heat and light for later use.

Carminative Tea

To help relieve the bloated, gaseous feeling associated with eating some foods, try this tea.

> 1 teaspoon dill or fennel seeds
> 1 teaspoon dried peppermint
> 1 cup boiling water

Bruise or crush the seeds with a mortar and pestle. If you don't have a mortar and pestle, put the seeds in a sealable plastic bag and hit them with a wooden mallet or rolling pin. Pour the seeds and peppermint into a cup or mug. Add boiling water. Cover and let steep for 15 to 20 minutes. Strain, then sip slowly.

Dill Casserole Bread

This bread recipe not only contains dill seeds to soothe upset stomachs, but also cottage cheese to boost your calcium intake. It's delicious, too.

1 tablespoon active dry yeast
¼ cup warm water
1 cup low-fat cottage cheese,
    at room temperature
2 tablespoons sugar
2 tablespoons melted butter, divided

2 tablespoons dill seeds
1 teaspoon salt
¼ teaspoon baking soda
1 large egg
1 cup whole-wheat flour
1½ cups unbleached all-purpose flour

1. Dissolve the yeast in the warm water and set aside.
2. In a mixing bowl, combine the cottage cheese, sugar, 1 tablespoon melted butter, dill seeds, salt, baking soda, and egg, beating until well blended. Stir in the softened yeast.
3. Add the whole-wheat flour and 1 cup of the unbleached flour. Gradually add remaining unbleached flour to form a stiff dough. Cover and let rise in a warm place for about 1 hour.
4. Stir the dough down and turn into a well-greased 8-inch round casserole dish (1½-quart size). Cover and let the dough rise 30 to 40 minutes.
5. Preheat the oven to 350°F (175°C) and bake the loaf for 35 to 45 minutes. Brush the top with the remaining melted butter. Let rest for 10 minutes before removing from the casserole dish to a rack to cool.

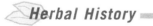 **Herbal History**

- Wild cats such as lions and tigers are affected by catnip in much the same way as their domesticated house cat cousins.
- Fennel seeds are crushed and applied to snakebites in China.
- Herbs mentioned in the Bible include dill and mint.

Woman's Care Garden

Whenever I give a lecture or class, I am struck by the number of women seeking information on herbs that will help them with problems specific to females. These plants are beautiful when grouped together, and will provide women with some of the remedies they seek.

CONTAINER GARDEN

This garden features potted herbs in willow or twig baskets of the appropriate size, placed in front of ground-planted fennel. One container holds the lemon balm and chamomile plants, the other contains the red clover. You can place Spanish moss on the surface and edges of each container that is nested in its basket to blend the edges. A special piece of statuary between the containers and the fennel will enhance the serenity of this spot.

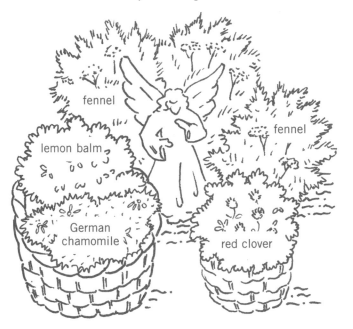

Container Garden Plants

- 3 fennel
- 1 lemon balm
- 7 German chamomile
- 1 red clover

PLOT GARDEN

Another idea is to set a rustic trellis behind the fennel to provide support and decoration; plant the other herbs in front of the fennel. This bed could be bordered by grapevines. You can achieve a twining effect by twisting together lengths of freshly cut grapevines. Move the vines into a desired shape and fasten into the ground with long metal staples to outline the herb bed.

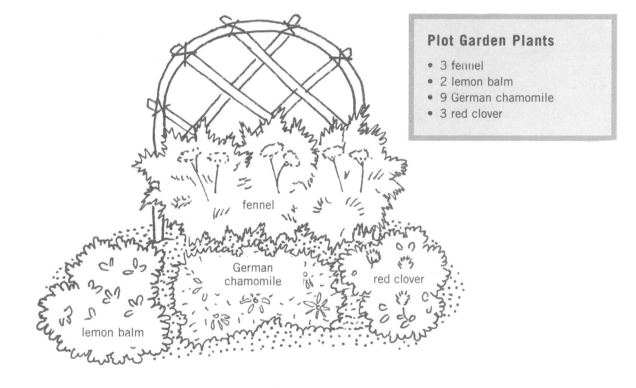

Plot Garden Plants

- 3 fennel
- 2 lemon balm
- 9 German chamomile
- 3 red clover

WOMAN'S CARE RECIPES

Women have different needs that must be addressed in the various stages of their lives. These simple recipes will take care of some of these needs.

Monthly Relief Tea

Drinking this infusion will help relieve menstrual cramps, but take no more than 2–3 cups a day.

  2 teaspoons dried lemon-balm leaves
  1 cup boiling water

Steep the leaves in the boiling water, covered, for 10 to 15 minutes. Strain, then slowly sip the infusion.

Dual-Purpose Tea

Sipping this infusion will relieve nausea and stomach upset, and lessen menstrual cramps. Do not drink more than 2 cups a day.

  2 teaspoons dried German chamomile flowers
  1 cup boiling water

Steep the flowers in the boiling water, covered, for 15 minutes. Strain, then slowly sip the infusion.

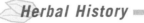

Herbal History

- Lemon balm is an ingredient in several liqueurs.
- Fennel was thought to aid weight loss because it has "skinny" leaves.
- Essential oil of chamomile is frequently an ingredient in perfumes.

Woman's Red Clover Tonic

This infusion, when sipped, will act as a tonic specially suited for women.

    1 teaspoon dried red clover blossoms
    1 cup boiling water

Add the blossoms to the boiling water. Cover and steep for 15 minutes. Strain, then sip the infusion.

Nursing Mother's Tea

Drinking a tea made with fennel helps to promote the secretion of breast milk in nursing mothers.

    1 teaspoon crushed fennel seeds
    1 cup boiling water

Mix the seeds with the boiling water. Cover and steep for 10 minutes. Strain, and sip the infusion.

ADDING RED CLOVER SPROUTS TO YOUR DIET

Red clover seeds can be sprouted and the sprouts used as a vitamin-packed addition to salads or sandwiches.

To sprout, use only organic seeds purchased for sprouting. Place about 1 tablespoon seeds in a quart jar and cover with clean water. Let the seeds soak for several hours or overnight. Drain the water off the seeds and cover the opening of the jar with cheesecloth or muslin. Rinse the seeds twice a day until the sprouts are ready to use with clean water and drain thoroughly. Store the jar on its side after each draining.

The sprouts can be used after they have grown an inch or two. They may be stored for several days in the refrigerator after they have sprouted.

Windowsill Medicine Cabinet

*T*he herbs in this collection can most easily be grown and maintained for fresh winter use in your home, making available to you a range of herbal treatments for a variety of complaints year-round. All of these plants will do best in east-, south-, and/or west-facing windows. Be aware that with less light available in winter, the plants could have a tendency to get leggy.

CONTAINER GARDEN #1

Plant each herb in its own container, choosing a different-sized and -shaped container for each; be sure each herb has enough growing space and a container that adds visual interest. Place the plants at windows throughout your house — wherever you have space.

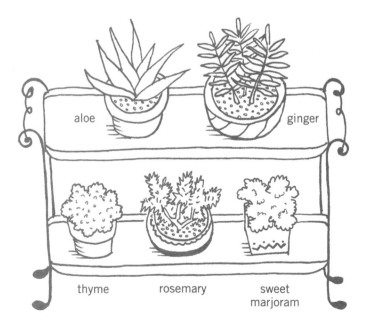

aloe   ginger

thyme   rosemary   sweet marjoram

Plants for Container Garden #1

- 1 aloe
- 1 ginger rhizome
- 1 thyme
- 1 rosemary
- 1 sweet marjoram

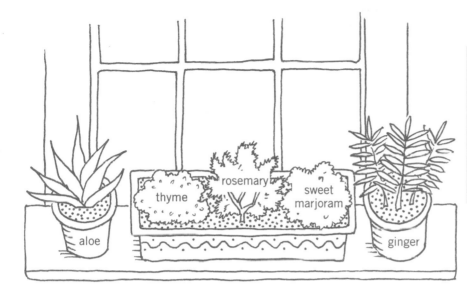

CONTAINER GARDEN #2

For a variation, put one plant each of thyme, rosemary, and sweet marjoram in a narrow trough that will fit on your windowsill. On either side of this trough, place a container of ginger and one of aloe.

Yet another plan calls for placing the Windowsill Medicine Cabinet in the windows of your potting shed and garage, as well as your house. Press metal shelving units or the steps of small ladders into service for multiple container plantings if your windows become overloaded. A large tray covered with 1 inch of gravel can be placed on the kitchen countertop next to a window with individually potted herbs in it.

Herbal History

- Rosemary has insect repellent qualities.
- Some of the herbs mentioned in Shakespeare's writings include chamomile, lavender, marjoram, mint, parsley, rosemary, and thyme.
- Sprigs of rosemary were once used to protect against the plague.
- Monasteries grew medicinal herbs in gardens next to their infirmaries.

WINDOWSILL MEDICINE CABINET RECIPES

All of the herbs in this garden, with the exception of aloe, can be used for culinary purposes.

Ginger Honey

Some herbal preparations aren't very palatable, but this one makes up for them. One teaspoon of the ginger honey may be taken for indigestion, gas, or nausea no more than three times a day. The ginger honey may also be substituted for the usual sweetener in your cup of tea.

¼ cup grated fresh ginger
1 cup honey

Place the honey and the ginger in a heatproof container such as a glass measuring cup. In a saucepan, pour 1–2 inches of water. Place the container in the water. Bring the water to a boil over high heat, then turn down to medium. Simmer for 30 minutes. Add more water if needed; do not let the water boil dry or the honey will scorch. After 30 minutes remove from the heat and allow to cool while still in the water. After cooling, strain the honey into a glass jar, label the jar, and store.

Sore Muscle Soak

This soak can be used in the bath for overall muscle soreness or in a basin to soak your sore, tired feet. For a bath, add the infusion and the bag of herbs to your bath water then soak in the tub until the water starts to feel cool. For a foot soak, pour the infusion into a basin. Add an additional 2 quarts of warm water. Soak your feet until the solution is cool.

2 tablespoons fresh or 1 tablespoon dried sweet marjoram
1 tablespoon fresh or 2 teaspoons dried rosemary
Muslin bath bag or old clean sock
1 quart water

Place the herbs in the bath bag or sock and fasten. Bring the water to a boil in an enamel or stainless-steel saucepan; add the herbs. Simmer for 10 minutes. Remove from the stove and allow the infusion to cool to lukewarm.

CHAPTER 6

Starting and Nurturing Your Plants

I f you browse through a catalog or go to a plant nursery to buy individual herb plants, you may become dismayed at how much money you have to spend to get all the plants you want and need. You can stretch your gardening budget farther by propagating your own herb plants.

There are different ways to increase the number of herb plants you have. All are relatively easy and require a minimum investment in equipment and supplies. I will discuss all of these different methods in detail.

STARTING HERB PLANTS FROM SEEDS

If you can obtain seeds for the herbs you want, it will be very economical for you to get a large quantity of plants. Herbs that can be started from seeds are calendula, catnip, cayenne, chamomile, dill, echinacea, fennel, feverfew, lavender, lemon balm, parsley, red clover, rosemary, sage, sweet marjoram, thyme, valerian, and yarrow.

Equipment for Starting Seeds

Equipment needs for seed starting are flexible. You will need trays or flats to hold pots or containers, small pots, clean empty yogurt containers, or reusable seed-starting kits that have a tray and "cells" to plant your seeds in. All containers should have holes in the bottom to promote drainage. The peat pots available on the market will also work as containers, but you must tear their sides and bottoms before planting them in the ground. The peat used to form these pots is so compacted and dense that roots cannot break through it. A sprinkling can and small bottle sprayer that can be filled with water are also needed, but the only tools you will require are your hands.

All containers must be extremely clean to prevent any diseases from being transferred to the soil and plants. To sterilize pots and containers, soak them in a 10 percent bleach solution (1 part bleach to 9 parts water) for 15 minutes. Let them dry thoroughly before using.

Let Them Have Light

A strong direct light source is essential for little seedlings. Some seeds need light to germinate, too. Inexpensive shop-light-type fixtures work well. Install one cool white fluorescent light tube and one warm white fluorescent light tube in each fixture. Suspend the lights about 3 inches away from the tops of the seedlings. You'll have to adjust these lights upward as the plants grow; don't let them touch the lights. Leave the lights on for 14 to 16 hours a day.

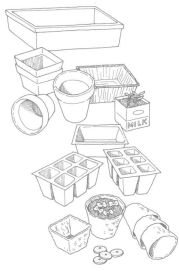

When you start herbs from seeds, you'll need a variety of trays, pots, and containers.

Starting the Seeds

Fill your chosen containers with the seed-starting mix. Don't pack the mix into the containers tightly — the seeds will have to struggle to grow any roots if the mix is compacted. Just scoop the containers into the mix and shake them, to settle the mix and eliminate any air pockets.

It is easy to get some of the little seedlings confused with each other, so use a waterproof marker to write the name of each herb on a piece of tape, and affix to the container. Sprinkle two or three seeds into each container or cell on top of the mix. Press the seeds lightly into the mix. Check the seed packages for seeds that require light to germinate; these should be pressed lightly into the soil. If the seeds need to be covered, a good rule of thumb is to add a depth of soil that is one to two times the size of the seed — which isn't a very great amount of soil. Covering them more deeply, however, could cause the seeds to rot before they sprout.

Soil that dries and forms a crust on seeds can prevent seedlings from emerging. There are a couple of ways to avoid this. One is to lightly mist the soil surface daily to keep it moist. The other is to cover the seeds not with soil but with vermiculite, which won't crust over.

Cover the containers of newly planted seeds with plastic wrap, window glass, or the plastic cover that comes with seed-starting kits. Keep them in a warm place (night temperatures of 60°–65°F, or 16°–18°C; day temperatures of 70°–75°F, or 21°–24°C) under lights and check daily for emerging seedlings. When these do emerge, remove the clear covering. Lightly mist the new seedlings with water occasionally. Keep the soil moist but do not overwater, because this would encourage fungal diseases. Lightly spraying the surface of the soil will accomplish this without dislodging the seeds. Allow the soil to dry out between waterings but do not allow the plants to wilt.

Special Seed Treatments: Stratification

Some seeds require special treatment to help them get started. One is stratification, which helps seeds break their dormancy. It involves exposing the seeds to cold, moist conditions — the kind they would encounter if they were to drop to the ground in fall, then spend winter on the cold and wet soil before the warmth of spring caused them to sprout.

You can mimic these conditions in your home easily. Place some moist vermiculite in a resealable plastic bag. Add whatever seeds require stratification; use one bag for each variety of seed. Expel as much air from the bag as you can, then close it. Label the bag and place it in your refrigerator for 2 months. I then take the vermiculite-seed mixture

STARTING MIXES

There are lots of seed-starting mixes available to put in your containers, or you can mix your own. Garden soil is too compact and can carry over diseases, so it isn't a good choice for seed starting. I like a light, well-draining commercial seed-starting mix with a few handfuls of vermiculite added.

Add water to moisten your seed-starting mix. Make the mix moist enough to feel damp but not so moist that you can squeeze water from it. I like to describe the feel of adequately moist seed-starting mix as the same as that of a moist cake.

and place it atop some seed-starter mix in small containers, which I treat just like the rest of the seeds I have planted. Echinacea and valerian seeds both require stratification. (Remember to stratify and start some of the endangered echinacea varieties such as *Echinacea pallida*. This will help increase the populations of plants that are dwindling due to overharvest and/or land development.)

Special Seed Treatments: Presprouting

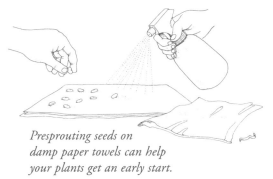

Presprouting seeds on damp paper towels can help your plants get an early start.

Presprouting seeds can get your plants off to an extra-early start. Dampen a couple of layers of paper toweling, and sprinkle some seeds on it. Roll up the paper towels and place them in a resealable plastic bag. Label the bag. Expel as much air from the bag as you can, then close it tightly. Place the bag in a warm spot (the top of your hot-water heater is excellent). After a few days have passed, check the seeds.

When they have started to sprout, carefully remove each fragile sprouted seed from the paper toweling and plant it in its own container with the same moisture and light as your other started seeds. Cover the sprouts lightly with a very thin layer of potting mix or vermiculite. If you can't remove the sprouts from the paper toweling without damaging them, tear a piece of the paper towel attached to each sprout and plant it, too. It will eventually degrade and will cause no harm to the plant. I find presprouting especially helpful in getting cayenne pepper plants started.

Special Seed Treatments: Presoaking

Some herbal literature mentions that parsley seeds should be presoaked, then the water discarded before the seeds are planted. Apparently the seeds have a natural coating that slows their germination. Although this may be true, I have not found that presoaking parsley seeds hastens their germination rate. Feel free to try it; perhaps your results will be different from mine.

Presoak seeds by placing them in room temperature water in an open container. Let the seeds soak overnight, then drain off the water and plant the seeds.

TESTING SEEDS FOR VIABILITY

Presprouting seeds serves another purpose, too: It helps you check old seeds for germination. Take any old seeds and sprinkle them on a damp paper towel, treating them as I described in presprouting. After a few days, unwrap the seeds and check to see how many have sprouted. This will help you to see approximately what percentage of seeds are viable and will sprout for you when you plant them. Take the presprouted seeds and plant them as described, or plant them directly into a prepared bed, covering them lightly.

Direct-Seeding

Planting seeds into the ground is simple, and appropriate for many plants. Some herbs grow easily when sown into the beds where they will spend the growing season. Prepare the soil and scatter the seeds widely where you want them to grow. Mixing the seeds with sand before planting will help you distribute them more widely. Use a garden rake to lightly scratch the seeds into the soil. Follow the directions on the seed packet, and if you cover the seeds, be sure to keep the seedbed moist enough that the soil doesn't crust over and prevent the new seedlings from breaking though. Thin new seedlings until there is appropriate space between them. Herbs that can easily be direct-seeded into your garden are calendula, catnip, dill, fennel, feverfew, German chamomile, lemon balm, sweet marjoram, and yarrow.

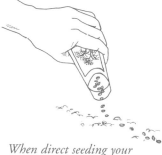

When direct seeding your herbs in an outdoor bed, be sure to space the seeds properly.

CARING FOR NEW SEEDLINGS

After your newly planted seeds sprout and grow in the ground, it is time to thin them so they'll have enough space to grow. This can be a painful project — it doesn't seem right to pull out plants that you have taken the trouble to grow. In fact, an old saying tells us to have someone else thin our seedbeds for us. If you don't have someone to do this task for you, then take a deep breath and do it yourself. Remember that the adult plants will need some space to grow without being crowded.

The act of thinning is simple. After your seedlings are two to three inches tall, pull out any seedlings that are stunted, damaged, or have misshapen leaves. Pull out the misshapen ones first, for it is unlikely that they will grow into healthy adult plants.

Dividing the Plants

When your new seedlings have grown enough to have a couple of sets of leaves, it is time to divide and/or thin them. If you have only two to three plants per container and the container is large enough to accommodate a growing plant, then remove the smaller plants, leaving the largest. You could transplant these culled plants into other containers if you want, or put them on your compost pile. The extra seedlings could also be cut off; put the cuttings on your compost pile. If you have several new seedlings in a small container, remove the clump of seedlings and transplant each into a larger container.

Separate the seedlings using a wooden tongue blade or plant marker as a miniature trowel. I usually start the seeds in small "cell packs" and transfer one plant each to a yogurt container. These containers are usually large enough to accommodate a growing herb plant until it is time to move into the ground or a larger container.

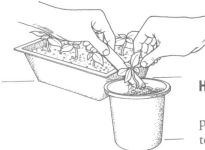

Use a wooden tongue blade to divide new seedlings for transplantation.

Watch your transplanted herbs. If you see roots growing from the bottom of the container it is time to move the plant into a larger container, or to transplant it outside if conditions are favorable.

Hardening

When the days start to warm and lengthen, it's time to toughen up your baby plants for their life outdoors. Do this gradually. The best place to start is in a sheltered shaded spot on a quiet day when the temperature is 55°F (13°C) or higher. Keep in mind that any wind, strong sunlight, or intense heat will be stressful to young plants. Leave them out for 15 to 30 minutes the first day, and gradually increase the time outside by 30 to 60 minutes each subsequent day.

Do not take your new plants outside on windy days. Tender young plants can have the life sucked from them by the wind. Keep a close eye on the weather. Bring your plants in if strong winds, below-freezing temperatures, or severe weather develops.

Transplanting and Spacing

You have now started your plants and acclimated them to the conditions outside. It is time to plant them into your herb beds and/or containers. Wait for the soil to warm and the weather to settle. Tender herbs must not go outside until after your frost-free date. Your local County Extension Service office can tell you this date if you don't know it. Pick a quiet day to plant them outside in their permanent location; a cloudy day with no gusty winds is ideal.

The soil should not be too wet to work in. To test it, squeeze a handful. If it forms a firm ball that does not break apart easily, then the ground is too wet to work in. If the soil doesn't form a firm ball easily, or if the ball breaks apart easily when touched, then it is ready for planting.

Decide how far apart you want to plant your herbs and dig a hole that is twice as wide and an inch or two deeper than the container that the herb is in. Loosen the soil inside the hole with a garden trowel to make it easier for your new herb plant's roots to grow. This is also a good time to work in compost or other soil amendments. Remove the plant from its container by holding it gently by the part of the stem that emerges from the soil, then squeezing or tapping the container to remove the plant along with most of the soil around its roots. Place the plant in the prepared hole, cover the rootball with soil, and firm it, leaving no air pockets. Hold the stem of the plant upright until you have enough soil around its roots to support it and keep it erect on its own. Water the plant well.

DAMPING OFF

Damping off is a fungal disease that affects newly emerged seedlings. You will see the stems of your new baby plants wilt, shrivel up, and fall over where the stem emerges from the soil. Should this occur, remove the affected plants and the soil mix they were in. Make sure that any plants near the affected ones are getting good air circulation and good drainage to prevent further occurrences of damping off.

When planting your herbs, include enough space between them so they can expand to their full size. See the Planting and Light Requirements chart for information on how large to expect your herb plants to be when they are mature.

STARTING HERBS FROM CUTTINGS

Stem cuttings will give you a new plant with the same characteristics as the mother plant. They are a good way to propagate and renew plants that are getting old. They're also a good way to propagate plants that won't grow true to seed or whose seeds have poor germination rates.

I know people who can start cuttings with the greatest of ease, but I have variable success with them. Some people can't seem to start them at all; all they end up with are containers of wilted stems and no new plants. Even those who propagate stem cuttings on a large scale don't have total success. I did some work with the groundskeeper at a retirement home one spring. They have a greenhouse there and grow most of their own plants. When I told him that I usually had only a 50 percent success rate with cuttings, he told me that that isn't so bad. Try to take your successes and failures in stride. Just be sure to start far more cuttings than you will need.

Starting the Cuttings in Soil

Prepare clean containers and a light seed-starting mix. I find that straight vermiculite works well. You will also need clean, sharp scissors. Some people use rooting hormone powder to stimulate root growth on cuttings. Others root their cuttings without the rooting hormone powder and have good success. I leave it up to you to decide whether or not you want to use it.

To start cuttings, chose strong, nonwoody growth. Late spring to early fall is a good time to take stem cuttings, since your plants have had the time to grow in optimal conditions. The long, leggy growth from winter months will not give you strong stem cuttings. Cut 3 to 6 inches off the chosen stem just below where leaves emerge from the stem, called a leaf node. The stem can be cut at an angle or straight across.

Strip half the leaves from each of your cuttings and remove any blooms. If you choose to use rooting hormone powder, pour a small amount of it on a piece of paper. Coat the half of the stem with no leaves by rolling it into the rooting hormone and tapping off the excess. Insert the lower half of your cuttings into your potting medium. Firm the mix around the stems, making sure there are no air pockets. Several cuttings can be inserted into a container 10 inches across or larger. Just be sure that the cuttings don't touch each other.

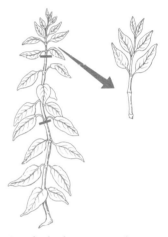

Cut the herb stem straight or at an angle.

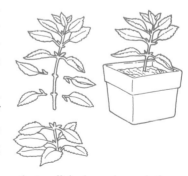

Strip off the lower leaves before transplanting the cutting.

Place them in a warm spot out of direct light. Lightly mist the cuttings twice a day with room-temperature water. Do not overwater; the soil should be kept damp but not waterlogged. Be patient. It will take several weeks for roots to form. You will know that the cuttings have taken root when a plant resists being pulled up with gentle tugging and/or there is new top growth.

Rooting Cuttings in Water

My grandmother's windowsill was full of little jelly glasses of water with plant cuttings in them. After a time I would see the water in the glasses full of little roots. Several years ago, starting cuttings in water fell out of favor; the thought was that the plants started this way were weak and did not grow as well. Now rooting cuttings in water has come back.

Take cuttings as I outlined above. Strip the leaves off the bottom third of the plant. Place the stripped part of the cuttings in a small container of water. Change the water in the container daily, and pot up your cuttings when they show vigorous root growth. Appearance of roots will vary according to the variety of plant.

PROPAGATING LIVE PLANTS

You have the potential to fit new herb plants in your existing garden. I will outline some ways to increase your herb plant population from existing plants in this section.

Layering

Some plants — such as thyme and mint — have stems that take root wherever they touch the ground. Others will need your help to form roots by layering.

Layering your plants requires less equipment and time than any other propagation method. The new plant forms while still attached to the mother plant, so the stem still obtains food and life strength from its plant of origin. Herbs to propagate in this way include peppermint, rosemary, thyme, and sage.

Select from the outer part of the mother plant a stem that will easily bend and touch the ground. Strip away any leaves from the section of stem that touches the soil, or take a knife and scrape away (or "wound") the outer coating of a small section of the stem. Dig and loosen the soil where the stem section touches. Anchor the stem into the soil using wire pins; you can make these from lengths of fence wire or large paper clips. Two pins, one on each side of the stem wound, should be sufficient. Bury the wounded section an inch or two into the soil. Water well, and lay a small stone or brick over the spot to anchor the layering and help retain moisture.

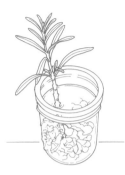

Cuttings can be placed in a glass or jar of water; transplant to pots when they show vigorous root growth.

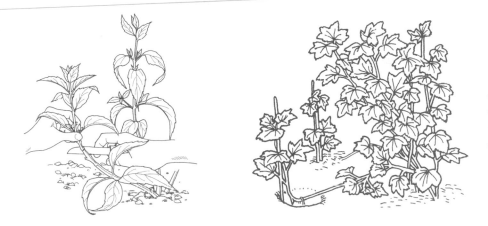

To propagate by layering, wound the selected plant stem by stripping the leaves and scraping off the outer stem coating (left). Anchor the wounded part of the stem to the soil with wire pins (right).

Layering can be accomplished in spring, summer, or fall. In spring or summer, it should take 6 to 8 weeks for roots to form; in fall, you will have to wait until the next spring for the appearance of new roots.

Check for new roots by carefully digging down into the soil around the area that you have layered. After new roots have formed, cut the layered stem from the mother plant and move it to a new spot in the garden or in a container.

Propagating Herbs by Division

When you are growing a lot of perennial herbs, you will find that dividing them is a good way to obtain more plants. It also is a good way to renew perennial herbs that have been around for a while and are nearing the end of their usefulness. Herbs that can be propagated by division include aloe, catnip, echinacea, fennel, lemon balm, mint, thyme (especially the low-growing varieties), valerian, and yarrow.

The ideal time to divide is in spring or fall. Use the divisions you pot up to sell or give away, or as container plantings. Increase the populations of divided plants by transplanting them directly into new places in your gardens.

To propagate by dividing, lift the mother plant in its entirety (or, if it's quite large, only a portion) with a garden fork. Shake the soil from the roots. Look at the plant that you have lifted for natural divisions. The divisions should have some roots and one or two stems coming from them. Pull the plant apart to divide, or cut apart with a knife or pruners if the clump is tightly woven. In older plants you can remove divisions from around the woody middle and take the woody part to your compost pile.

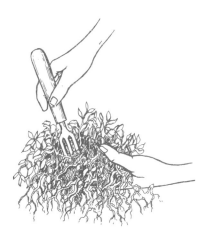

Examine the dug up herb clump for natural divisions, and gently pull apart.

Water the divisions thoroughly and trim some of the top growth. Leaving too much top growth will cause the new division to lose moisture. Keep the new plantings well watered. Watch for new growth, a sign that your plant is established.

Planting and Light Requirements

Plant size will ultimately depend on the growing conditions that the herb is exposed to. The following information will give you an idea of what to expect from your herbs. To fill out a space more quickly, you can plant your herbs closer together than is listed; just don't overcrowd them.

HERB	ADULT HEIGHT	SPACING
Aloe	1–2 feet (30–60 cm)	1 foot (30 cm) apart
Calendula	6–12 inches (15–30 cm), depending on variety	8–12 inches (20–30 cm) apart
Catnip	1–3 feet (30–90 cm)	6–12 inches (15–30 cm) apart
Cayenne	1–2 feet (30–60 cm)	2 feet (60 cm) apart
Dill	3–4 feet (.9–1.2 m)	8–10 inches (20–25 cm) apart
Echinacea	2–3 feet (60–90 cm)	8–10 inches (20–25 cm) apart
Fennel	4–5 feet (1.2–1.5 m)	8–12 inches (20–30 cm) apart
Feverfew	2–3 feet (60–90 cm)	8–12 inches (20–30 cm) apart
Garlic	1–3 feet (30–90 cm)	3–6 inches (7.5–15 cm) apart
German chamomile	2 feet (60 cm)	8 inches (20 cm) apart
Ginger	2–4 feet (.6–1.2 m)	1 foot (30 cm) apart
Lavender	14–24 inches (35–60 cm), depending on variety	1½–2 feet (46–60 cm) apart
Lemon balm	2 feet (60 cm)	1–2 feet (30–60 cm) apart
Parsley	12–18 inches (30–46 cm)	6–12 inches (15–30 cm) apart
Peppermint	2–3 feet (60–90 cm)	6 inches (15 cm) apart
Red clover	2 feet (60 cm)	1½–2 feet (46–60 cm) apart
Rosemary	2–4 feet (.6–1.2 m)	2 feet (60 cm) apart
Sage	1–3 feet (30–90 cm)	18–20 inches (46–50 cm) apart
Sweet marjoram	1–2 feet (30–60 cm)	6–8 inches (15–20 cm) apart
Thyme	3–12 inches (7.5–30 cm), depending on variety	6–12 inches (15–30 cm) apart
Valerian	3–5 feet (.9–1.5 m)	2 feet (60 cm) apart
Yarrow	3 feet (90 cm)	1 foot (30 cm) apart

TYPE OF PLANT	LIGHT REQUIREMENTS	SPECIAL CONSIDERATIONS
tender perennial	full sun to partial shade	grow as a container plant
annual	full sun	self-seeds
perennial	full sun to partial shade	will grow in poor soil
annual	full sun	wear gloves when handling fruit to avoid skin irritation
annual	full sun	do not plant near fennel because of cross-pollination
perennial	full sun to partial shade	good to use in butterfly gardens
perennial	full sun	do not plant next to dill because of cross-pollination
perennial	full sun to partial shade	self-seeds
annual	full sun to partial shade	fall plant; cover with mulch
annual	full sun to partial shade	self-seeds
tender perennial	partial shade	grow as a container plant
perennial	full sun	different varieties are appropriate for different growing areas
perennial	full sun to partial shade	self-seeds
biennial	full sun to partial shade	slow germination of seeds when planted
perennial	full sun to partial shade	has invasive tendencies; will tolerate wet soil
biennial	full sun	self-seeds
tender perennial	full sun to partial shade	grow in containers in cold-weather climates to avoid trauma to the roots when transplanting
perennial	full sun	semievergreen foliage in winter
tender perennial	full sun	warmth and full sun are necessary for essential-oil production
perennial	full sun	thrives in poor soil; semievergreen foliage in winter
perennial	full sun to partial shade	self-seeds
perennial	full sun	self-seeds

Propagating Herbs

HERB	GERMINATION REQUIREMENTS			PROPAGATION METHOD			
	REQUIRE LIGHT	DON'T REQUIRE LIGHT	PRESPROUTING RECOMMENDED	DIVISION	LAYERING	STEM CUTTINGS	REQUIRE STRATIFICATION
Aloe				X			
Calendula		X					
Catnip		X		X		X	
Cayenne		X	X				
Dill	X						
Echinacea		X		X			X
Fennel		X		X			
Feverfew		X					
Garlic		x; plant cloves					
German chamomile		X					
Ginger		x; plant rhizomes					
Lavender		X				X	
Lemon balm	X			X		X	
Parsley		X					
Peppermint				X	X	X	
Red clover		X					
Rosemary		x; variable germination			X	X	
Sage		X			X	X	
Sweet marjoram	x*				X		
Thyme	X			X	X	X	
Valerian		X		X			X
Yarrow		X		X			

*recommended, but not absolutely necessary

CHAPTER 7

Garden Maintenance

arden maintenance includes feeding, watering, trimming, and weeding your herbs. Most of us have less time for our hobbies and pursuits than we would like, so planning and planting your garden for low maintenance is the best idea, particularly if you are a first-time gardener.

If you prepared your soil well, thoroughly digging in lots of organic matter, then your first step toward easy maintenance has been taken. Soil with lots of organic matter will drain better and provide nutrients to your herb plants. Well-fed plants will be more resistant to pests and diseases.

PLOT GARDEN MAINTENANCE

Certain tasks, when performed, can keep your garden looking good throughout the growing season. This section tells you what those tasks are, but don't feel that you are obligated to perform each one of them. Herbs are resilient — if you don't get around to some of the maintenance, they will forgive you.

Trimming and Deadheading

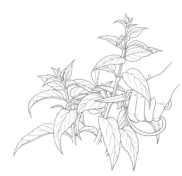

Gardening scissors or hand pruners should be used to trim herb plants to the desired height and shape.

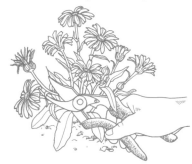

To prevent plants from self-seeding, deadhead them by cutting off spent blossoms.

Some herb plants can become tall and overgrown; this can look unkempt. Trimming herb plants with gardening scissors or hand pruners can both give them a more pleasing shape and provide you with fresh herbs to use. When trimming, cut the stem to the desired height; make this cut just above where a set of leaves comes out of the stem. Cutting here should encourage the plant to branch out and become bushier. Removing selected stems will prevent crowding in bushy herbs. Herbs that can benefit from a shapely trimming are catnip, feverfew, lemon balm, peppermint, rosemary, sage, and thyme. Don't discard the healthy parts that you remove; harvest them instead.

Deadheading is the act of removing blooms that are past their prime. It serves several purposes. It removes unsightly spent blooms, making the plant more attractive. In many plants deadheading can encourage more blooming, helping to keep your herb garden in continuous bloom.

Deadheading prevents the plant from self-seeding and scattering new plants into places you don't want them. If, however, you would like more herbs of a certain variety without the work of planting, allow them to self-seed. You have to be willing to relocate seedlings that pop up in unwanted spaces, but the number of seedlings you can get from reseeding can be worth it. Herbs that self-seed easily include calendula, German chamomile, dill, echinacea, fennel, feverfew, lemon balm, red clover, thyme, and yarrow.

Trim herb plants as they need it and deadhead flowers as you desire. Harvest individual herbs as you want when they are ready. Remove and destroy diseased plants.

Watering

If you've added organic matter to your soil, it should hold enough moisture to provide your plants with the water they need. To check the soil for water, dig down 3 or 4 inches. If the soil is moist there, then the plants do not need watering. If the soil feels dry, then it's time to water.

Deep-watering is essential to help the plant grow a good root system. You can't easily accomplish this with a sprinkling can or hose, however; you'll need a sprinkler or soaker hose. If you use a sprinkler, bury a small open can in the ground with about one inch of the open end above ground level to measure the amount of water you're giving. Let the sprinkler run until the can has 1 to 1½ inches of water in it. To minimize evaporation of the water, you can bury a soaker hose in mulch for the growing season and use it to water plants. For a thorough watering, let the water run for about 4 to 6 hours to get adequate moisture to the roots of the herbs. Check your soil for moisture weekly — more frequently if it is very dry — and water if needed.

Avoid working in a wet garden. Moisture from diseased plants will spread these diseases from your hands and tools to other plants. Also, if you walk on wet garden soil you'll cause compaction, making it rock hard when it dries.

Weeding

A general definition of a *weed* is "any plant that pushes its way into a garden and is unwanted." Given this definition, weeds can be both those plants traditionally thought of as weeds, and any garden plants that have spread or self-seeded in unexpected places.

Weeding is most easily accomplished the day after you water or receive rainfall. This loosens the soil and makes it easier to pull weeds. For weeds with deep taproots, cut this taproot several inches below ground level if you can't pull it. Mulching will keep the growth of weeds down.

Fall Cleanup

After the first killing frost, pull out all of your dead annuals and take them to the compost pile if they were not diseased. I do not trim off any of my browned perennials in fall; the brown stalks help me locate the plants next spring before they start to green up again, along with giving the garden some character during the winter months. Not trimming the plants in fall will also help protect their crowns or center from moisture; trapped moisture inside the crown can freeze and kill the plants. Trim the perennials' dead stalks off to the level of new growth in the early warmth of spring when you see new growth beginning at ground level.

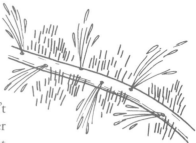

A soaker hose provides deep watering for healthy root growth.

GO EASY

When spring gives us longer, warmer days, I become enthusiastic. I find that I initially go out and work muscles that I haven't used for several months. The result is stiffness and soreness. Avoid this by initially working for just a short amount of time. Do some stretching exercises three to four times a week to help get your muscles conditioned. Get your body used to garden work gradually. If and when you overdo it, see the Sore Muscle Garden for ideas on how to take care of yourself. (See page 140.)

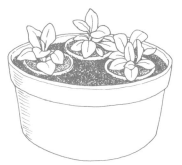

Container plantings are attractive decorations, as well as good ways to maintain a garden in cold weather or limited space.

CONTAINER GARDEN MAINTENANCE

Container planting has become very popular. It is a practical trend; some of us don't have a lot of land on which to plant gardens. The portability of containers makes it easy to move them around and place them on patios and decks as well as indoors. Containers placed on tables or other elevated spots are accessible to gardeners unable to bend over and tend a garden planted in the ground.

Containers can be the traditional clay pots or whatever unconventional items are available to you. There is a unique learning and life center near my home that sees usefulness in many items generally headed for the landfill. These folks take "junk" and incorporate it into one-of-a-kind plantings and gardening decorations. Train your mind to view such items as objects you could use in your gardening designs. Some examples of containers you can use are strawberry jars, coffee cans, olive-oil cans, hollowed-out logs, half barrels, and old sprinkling cans. The sky is the limit!

Condition the Container Plants

When it's time to bring your container plants inside in fall, do so gradually; the process is the reverse of hardening off plants in spring. Know where you're going to put the containers. Start a couple of weeks before the first frost and gradually increase the plants' time indoors in the space you have chosen.

You'll probably need to water frequently, because the humidity in your home is much less than that outside. Plants inside your house will also like an occasional misting, again because of the lower humidity. Sunlight and air circulation requirements are about the same as for outdoor plants. Go easy on trimming and harvesting herbs you've brought in for the cold months; harvest only as the plants develop more new growth. When warm weather returns, gradually take the plants back outside.

Container Gardens as Decoration

If you are the type of person who likes to rearrange things around your home, container plantings may be just the thing for you. You can move the containers around inside and outside for a new look.

You can also change the look of the containers themselves by placing them in baskets, pottery, or other objects. You don't have to replant — just slip the pot into the new container. When watering, be sure to empty the container of any standing water that drains out of the pot, or remove the potted plant for watering before returning it to its decorative cover.

Watering and Drainage

Any container you use must have good drainage. Make sure there are holes punched in the bottom to give plants that drainage. If containers are outside, I usually do not put them in dishes; during prolonged rainy spells the dishes hold water and give the plant the same wet conditions it would have if it were in a chronically wet spot in the ground.

Clay containers are porous and will lose moisture more quickly. If your climate tends to be dry, nonporous containers such as those made from plastic might be your best choice. They will help the soil to hold water longer.

Container plants will probably need more frequent watering than plants in the ground. Dig down an inch or two with your fingers or a small garden trowel into the soil to check for moisture. If there is none, it is time to water. Water container plantings from the top. Minerals from your water can accumulate in the soil of container plantings, creating a white coating on the top of the potting soil; watering from the top will help flush them out.

During very dry spells, container-grown herbs appreciate a light misting of water in the early-morning hours. It cleans the leaves and refreshes them. This is especially good for herbs and other plants grown indoors, where the humidity is lower.

Container Soil

Regular garden soil is not appropriate for container plantings regardless of what type you have. Regular soil is heavier than commercial potting mixes and will compact, hindering your plants' root growth. There are many potting mixtures available that are appropriate for container-grown herbs, though. Some of the less expensive mixes tend to be too heavy, but you can include combinations of additives to enhance their drainage capability, including peat, vermiculite, perlite, and compost.

Be sure to give new plants some space for their roots and foliage to grow in your chosen container. Overcrowding can invite pest and disease problems.

Sinking the Containers

Rather than disturbing the roots of plants that you plan to bring in come cold weather, sink a container of the chosen plants into the ground for the warm months so that they blend in with the rest of your garden. Dig a large hole and fit the container into it, leaving about 1 inch of the top rim above the ground level. Any herb can be planted this way, but it is especially good for tender perennials that you want to overwinter inside, and also helps to contain mints.

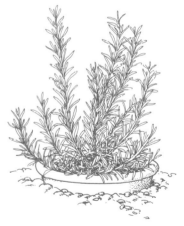

To save yourself time, sink container herbs into your outdoor gardens in the warmer months. They will be easy to dig up and transfer indoors when the temperature drops.

Light Requirements

Container plantings need the same amount of direct sunlight as plants in herb beds. You can move containers around during the day, however, to achieve their optimal amount of sunlight. If the container is heavy, place it on a platform with rollers for easy moving.

Clay pots exposed to direct sun in the hottest part of the day can become too hot. This can stress plants and even "fry" the roots of some of them. Positioning clay pots in dappled sunlight will help keep the heat to a minimum.

GARDENING LEFTOVERS

The following are some gardening tips and ideas that I have found useful. Read them over; perhaps they can help you, too, with special situations.

Finding the Perfect Spot

Plant herbs in a temporary spot and observe them for a season to get an idea of their growing shape and habit. This will help you decide where to grow each type of herb and how to plant it in relation to its herbal neighbors. I keep a separate bed dubbed "the holding bed" just for this purpose.

Once established, herbs will fill in a space. When you plant them, then, allow some room for them to grow and spread. If you want herbs to fill a space in a shorter amount of time, plant them closer together, but keep in mind that later in the season they can become crowded. Such overcrowding can lead to decreased air flow in among them, which can encourage diseases.

Decorative Planting

Add colorful annual or perennial flowers that are also considered to be herbs to your herb garden to lend bright color when you want it. Some choices are pansies, nasturtiums, bee balm, roses, carnations, and violets.

Taking a Vacation from Your Garden

Leaving your plants even for as little as a week requires some planning. Place container-grown plants in a shadier situation where they will not lose moisture quite as readily. Water everything thoroughly before you go. To give your plants some water while you are away, place one end of a thick cotton rope in a container of water, and the other end in the soil of the container you want watered. The rope acts as a wick, giving the plant a constant supply of moisture.

Container Gardens

To conserve moisture in containers, mulch the surface of the potting mix your plants live in. You can also add a special polymer additive for water retention, or you can add bentonite clay at a ratio of 1 part bentonite to 16 parts potting mix. Bentonite is a special clay found in natural food stores and homebrewing supply shops; it has a high capacity for absorbing and holding moisture.

"Tour the Grounds"

After a day of working on our gardens, my husband and I often do what we half jokingly call "touring the grounds." This involves walking around the property, admiring the plants and our hard work. We stop to look at any plant that is in bloom, pinch off some herbs to smell, and generally enjoy the results of our efforts. This is also a good time to look at the "big picture" of the property, seeing if things are planted in a pleasing way and planning for future projects and chores. We've come up with all kinds of ideas while strolling through our gardens. It also gives us a chance to take a deep breath and enjoy the place.

Take visitors to your home for a garden tour, too. Many people enjoy gardens but can't put forth all the effort needed to have one. Showing people around your gardens can be an opportunity for them to see herbs and learn about some of their uses. Having them admire your work can be a great boost to your ego as well! I have found most visitors to my gardens to be admiring as well as grateful for the learning experience.

Gardening is a pleasant pastime and good exercise. Always take a little time out from your work to enjoy the results of your care. I have spent some enjoyable moments admiring my gardens while taking a work break under a nearby tree. After you've gone through the work of planting a garden, make an effort to enjoy it. Sit out in or near the gardens and enjoy the sight and aroma while thinking about the usefulness of the herbs. It is a pleasant way to pass some time. You deserve it after making the effort of planning and planting!

Teaching Children about Herbs

Children seem to be intrigued by herbs, and it's to their benefit to get them involved in herb gardening if you can. I'm not sure if it is the aroma that draws them in, or the stories surrounding the herbs and their uses. Whatever the reason, children are very happy to be around plants that smell good — and that they have permission to touch and pick. It may surprise you to find out how much information about the herbs they remember.

WINDOW BOXES

In my opinion these are some of the most lovely containers around. You can permanently attach or temporarily hook boxes to the windows around your home. In either case, though, they must be attached in a sturdy manner because of the weight of the soil and plants they contain.

Soil requirements are as for other containers. Choose plants according to exposure to sun and rain from the direction that the plants will be best viewed. Cascading herbs such as prostrate rosemary or creeping thyme will look lovely planted to drape over the edge of the window boxes.

Whenever my son and I were around herbs together I would explain what each plant was and how it could be used, picking a bit for him to smell. I can still recall watching him — when he was very young — pointing out some herbs to his friend. "Do you see that plant?" he asked. "Guess what it's used for." Then he launched into an accurate explanation. I was pleased and a bit surprised.

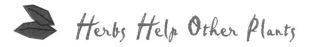

Herbs Help Other Plants

Besides their traditional uses, herbs can be planted among your vegetables to aid in their growth. Some gardeners swear by this, although some declare that the herbs do nothing to help other plants. Try planting a few in your vegetable garden to see if you notice a difference. To keep some of the more vigorous and invasive herbs from taking over your vegetable patch, plant them in containers placed among your vegetables.

HERB	BENEFITS TO OTHER PLANTS
Calendula	Repels tomato worms and carrot flies.
Catnip	Repels flea beetles, squash bugs, Japanese beetles, and aphids. Attracts honeybees.
Dill	Attracts beneficial insects.
Garlic	Repels aphids, cabbage worms, slugs, snails, Japanese beetles, and rabbits.
Lavender	Repels aphids.
Lemon balm	Attracts honeybees.
Peppermint	Attracts beneficial insects. Repels ants, aphids, flea beetles, squash bugs, and whiteflies.
Parsley	Attracts beneficial insects.
Rosemary	Repels bean beetles, cabbage moths, slugs, and snails.
Sage	Repels cabbage moths.
Thyme	Repels cabbage moths and whiteflies. Attracts honeybees.
Yarrow	Attracts beneficial insects.

Controlling Pests and Diseases

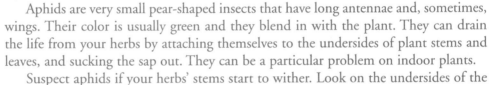

erbs in general seem to have minimal pest and disease problems. Some herbs, particularly garlic and cayenne pepper, are actually used as pest repellents. There are several nontoxic ways to deal with pests when and if they appear in your herb gardens. The use of chemical pesticides can present appreciable risks to land, water, and people. You must weigh the lasting effects of pesticides on your crops and land against their benefits against pests. It is your choice to make.

IDENTIFYING AND ELIMINATING PESTS

Despite most herbs' resistance to pests, there are some that manage to do some damage from time to time. It is to your advantage to be able to recognize them should your plants begin to develop problems. Proper identification will then help you to plan how to eradicate the pests and minimize the damage.

Aphids

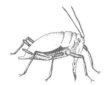

Aphid

Aphids are very small pear-shaped insects that have long antennae and, sometimes, wings. Their color is usually green and they blend in with the plant. They can drain the life from your herbs by attaching themselves to the undersides of plant stems and leaves, and sucking the sap out. They can be a particular problem on indoor plants.

Suspect aphids if your herbs' stems start to wither. Look on the undersides of the stems and leaves to find them. Another symptom of this pest is that you will feel stickiness on the leaves and stems. This is the aphids' excrement, called honeydew, and it will attract both ants and a mold that will color your plants black. To rid your plants of aphids, spray with an insecticidal soap or very fine horticultural oil, both of which can be found in gardening supply stores and catalogues. If aphids are a problem outdoors, plant nasturtiums near your herbs. Aphids are attracted to nasturtiums, which will act as a "trap crop" for the pests, drawing them away from other plants. Also, ladybugs and green lacewings will eat aphids.

Whiteflies

Whitefly

Whiteflies are small, light-colored winged insects that live indoors and out. Whiteflies and their young, called nymphs, are notorious pests in greenhouses, but they can also make an appearance in your house. Like aphids, whiteflies suck plant sap from leaves and stems. Suspect their presence if your herbs are withering and weakening. If the plants are brushed or otherwise disturbed, you'll see the adults flying around them. The nymphs will be on the undersides of plant stems and leaves.

Control whiteflies with an insecticidal soap spray or very fine horticultural oil spray. They can also be trapped on the yellow "sticky" traps found in garden supply stores; or you can smear petroleum jelly or a similar tenacious substance on a piece of yellow cardboard to trap them. A parasitic wasp called *Encarsia formosa* will kill whiteflies by laying eggs in the nymphs, but will not cause damage to the plants.

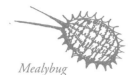

Mealybug

Mealybugs

Another pest common on plants grown indoors is the mealybug. Mealybugs look like little bits of white or yellowish cotton and are found on the undersides of plant leaves. They, too, suck sap from your plants and excrete honeydew. Suspect mealybugs if your plants are becoming withered and weak. The leaves might even look yellow.

Spraying your plants with a strong stream of water will knock these bugs off. If you have an infestation on just one or two plants, dip a cotton swab in rubbing alcohol and touch each mealybug with it to kill them. You can also try a spray solution of insecticidal soap or very fine horticultural oil spray. An insect called *Cryptolaemus montrouzieri* or lady bird beetle is available commercially for release in enclosed areas to control large mealybug infestations. The adults and larvae of this insect eat mealybugs, and cause no apparent damage to the plants.

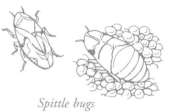

Spittle bugs

Spittle Bugs, Scale, and Spider Mites

Spittle bugs are easily identifiable. These sap-sucking insects are small and brown-green in color, but you probably won't see them. What you will see is a white frothy secretion that surrounds the insect. They are most commonly found on plant stems, often where a leaf attaches. The easiest way to evict spittle bugs from your plants is to spray them with a strong stream of water.

Scale is another sap-sucking pest. Small, oval, and brown to cottony white in color, scale can be found on the stems of plants. Affected plants will turn yellowish and show slowed or stunted growth. Dab each scale with a cotton swab dipped in rubbing alcohol or spray with a very fine horticultural oil spray solution to eradicate them.

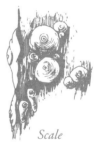

Scale

Spider mites are very tiny insects. They are almost too small to see, but you will notice their webs on your plants. Mainly an indoor pest, spider mites suck the juices from your plants. The leaves of your plants will curl, with little webs woven among their stems and leaves. You can confirm mites' presence by shaking a plant after putting a white piece of paper under it. Spider mites will fall on the paper — they will be dark and about the size of a grain of sand. Spray with a strong stream of water to evict them or use an insecticidal soap solution.

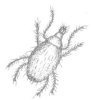

Spider mite

Japanese Beetles

Japanese beetle

Japanese beetles are found throughout the eastern United States. Just about everyone recognizes these greenish copper flying beetles and has seen the damage they cause as they chew on the leaves and flowers of a great number of plants, including herbs. Suspect Japanese beetles if you see great pieces of leaves between the veins chewed away and flowers missing or chewed on. You will probably see the beetles themselves on and around the plant. The white grubs found in your yard are the larvae of Japanese beetles. Controlling them will decrease the populations somewhat, but if your neighbors aren't controlling the grubs, you will still have the beetles visiting your plants.

The Japanese beetle traps so prevalent in peoples' yards nowadays will probably attract more beetles to your area than they will trap. The advice given jokingly in gardening classes is for you to buy your neighbor one of these traps! I know of a gardener who handpicks them from her plants, then "stomps on them." (I think the act of stomping makes her feel better.) Placing a large piece of canvas or plastic on the ground, shaking the infested plants, and dumping the beetles into a bucket of soapy water will help with localized infestations. Birds will also eat them, so encourage their visits to your garden with birdbaths and feeders.

Slugs and Snails

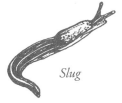

Slug

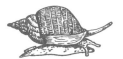

Snail

Slugs and snails are soft-bodied creatures in the mollusk family. They are slimy and gray to brown in color. Snails have coiled shells; slugs don't. Both love moist, dark places and come out at night to feast on plants. Suspect snails or slugs if you see sections of plants eaten away and silvery trails between plants made from the mucus they excrete.

There are several ways to control them. Because of their soft bodies, they do not like rough terrain, so surrounding your plants with a layer of wood chips, wood ashes, or sand will help deter them. Another way to battle slugs and snails is to use diatomaceous earth, a white powdery substance made from the fossilized shells of ancient tiny sea creatures called diatoms. Dust it on and around affected plants. The sharp edges of the diatom skeletons will pierce the soft bodies of the slugs and snails and cause death.

There is yet another method that works very well to rid your garden of slugs and snails: Fill empty tuna cans or jar lids with beer and leave them out by your plants. Slugs and snails like beer so much that they will literally drown in it. If you want to get personally involved in snail and slug eradication, try this. Arm yourself with a container of soapy water and a flashlight and go out in the garden after dark to pick slugs and snails off their plants, dumping them into the soapy water. Many gardeners do this with good results and apparently much satisfaction!

Deer

One animal universally mentioned as a pest by gardeners all over the United States is the deer. Mainly due to the lack of natural predators, there are more deer in the U.S. now than there were when Europeans first arrived. They can devastate a garden in a short time.

Deer will randomly eat herbs. They seem to leave some of the more aromatic herbs, at least in my gardens. These include thyme, lavender, and the mints.

There are many ideas on how to deter deer. Some work, and some don't. The fact is that if the deer are hungry enough, they will eat what they want. They like to have cover nearby in which to hide, so if you have a deer problem, try not to plant your herb beds next to a line of trees and bushes. Some gardeners sprinkle blood meal around plants to deter the animals. Others tie bars of deodorant soap throughout the garden. Some swear by spreading human hair around their gardens, saying that the odor will deter deer.

Covering your plants with netting will keep deer from eating your plants down to their stems. Regular fencing is not a deterrent. Deer can easily jump over 3- to 4-foot-high fences. Higher 6-foot-tall fences seem to keep them out. If deer are damaging to your garden, it is worth trying any of these deterrents. Stay flexible and change methods if the first one doesn't work.

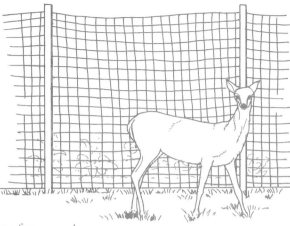

A tall fence is the best method of keeping deer out of your garden.

LET THE BENEFICIAL "PESTS" HELP YOU

Should you find your herb plants being eaten by an insect pest, do not take immediate action. Wait a day or two to see if any beneficial insects will step in to help eradicate pests for you. Many predator insects and their larvae will feed on pests. Examples are ladybugs, green lacewings, and praying mantids. Close observation will help you to learn which insects are helpful and which aren't.

Nematodes are tiny, hairlike creatures; there are different kinds of them, some harmful to the garden and others helpful. Some of the helpful ones battle different insects. One strain is parasitic on Japanese beetle grubs, feeding on the grubs then reproducing in their bodies. You can order these beneficial nematodes in garden specialty catalogs. (See Resources.)

Some companies sell predator insects. When they arrive, you turn them loose into your garden to eat harmful insects. It all sounds quite simple, but these bugs will not stay if they don't have the proper conditions in which to live and food to sustain them. Do your homework before buying them.

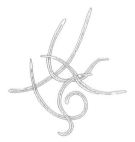

Beneficial nematodes prey on other insect pests such as Japanese beetles.

Besides the predators already mentioned, there are some other creatures in the garden that will help you with your crop — although you may not think of them as friends. Spiders and wasps will both eat insects in your garden and should be allowed to live there. Bumblebees are great crop pollinators and are more important now than ever, with the honeybee population in decline due to pests and disease. Toads are quite fond of insects; give them free rein in your garden. Bats, too, should be encouraged to live in your vicinity.

The last few years we have had a literal invasion of ladybugs into our house in fall. I have learned to let a few stay around. They don't hurt anything and will help to get rid of some of the pests that like indoor plants.

Beneficial insects are attracted to the flowers of parsley and fennel, so grow these herbs in your gardens to encourage them. Other herbs that beneficial insects like are red clover, calendula, and yarrow. I also leave Queen-Anne's-lace growing around the edge of my gardens; this plant's white umbel flowers attract beneficial insects, too.

Encourage birds to live near your gardens as well; many will eat insects. Birdhouses, -baths, and feeders can help attract them.

NONTOXIC INSECT DETERRENTS

I have mentioned a few substances used to combat insect pests in the garden that aren't toxic to humans or the environment. Inside your home, you can use insecticidal soap and very fine horticultural oil without fear of toxicity to humans or animals. Here is more information.

Diatomaceous earth. Made from the cracked fossilized shells of single-celled sea creatures call diatoms, this powdery white substance works by piercing the soft bodies of pests such as slugs and snails. Diatomaceous earth must be applied to the tops, undersides, or area surrounding affected plants that are moist from dew, rain, or watering to aid in sticking. Do not dust the flowers on a plant. Diatomaceous earth can harm some beneficial insects. Wear a filter mask when applying diatomaceous earth — the dust can be a lung irritant. Reapply it after a rain. I do not recommend using it in your house.

Insecticidal soap. This is not the same kind of soap you use for the household and bath. Insecticidal soap doesn't make suds. The fatty acids it contains act as a natural insecticide and seem to be most effective against soft-bodied insects such as aphids, mealybugs, spider mites, and whiteflies. Follow package directions for mixing and apply with a sprayer.

Horticultural oil. This substance, also known as paraffinic oil, is refined enough to spray on plants after the foliage has come on to control aphids, scale, mealybugs, and whiteflies. I have also found it to be effective against different caterpillar pests, yet harmless to beneficial insects. Follow package directions to mix the oil and apply with a sprayer.

...ract insect pests. Plants suit-
...ell fed and cared for are also
...nse when a plant is stressed;
...n in good shape with well-
...will go a long way toward
...getting rid of hiding places

...uate drainage, fertility, and
...hat can affect your herbs. As
...wer disease problems.

...around your plants, here is
...ing of green scum on it and
...ants to grow.

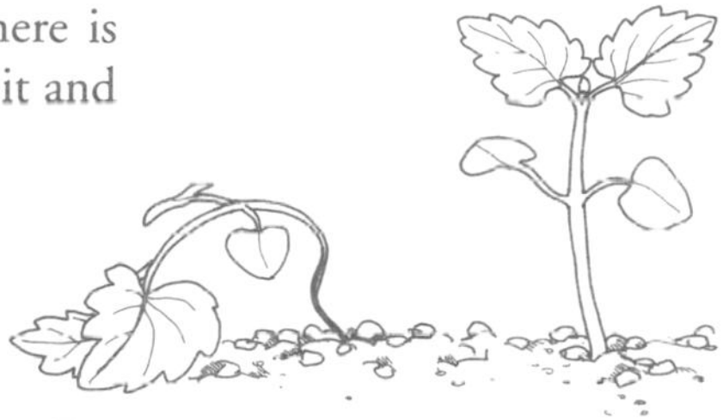

...ngs. It happens soon
...ey will become limp,
...troy the affected plants. Do
...e. To prevent damping off,
...nent. Don't overwater the
...off can occur with any herb
...the most susceptible.
...amomile or nettle tea (or a
...s. Water seedlings with tea

*Damping off disease destroys
seedlings by weakening them
shortly after emergence.*

until they are ready for transplantation.

Powdery mildew looks like a white fuzzy powder on plant leaves. The leaves will ultimately turn brown and drop off. Affected plants must be removed to avoid spreading the disease. To prevent powdery mildew, provide good drainage and air circulation to your plants. Full sunlight will help dry moisture from plants after a morning dew or rain. Keep your herbs trimmed for optimal air circulation. Calendula, lemon balm, rosemary, and yarrow are particularly susceptible to powdery mildew.

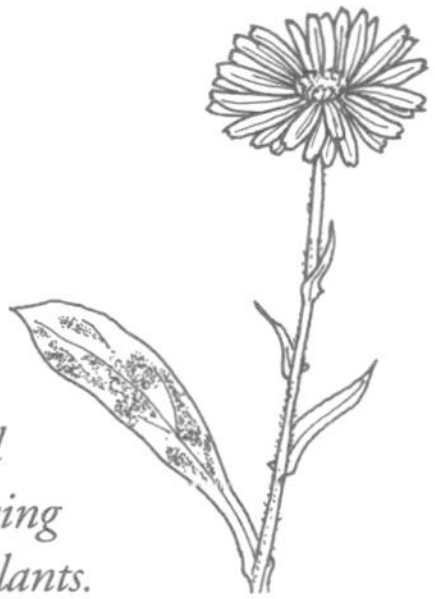

*Powdery
mildew
can only
be treated
by destroying
affected plants.*

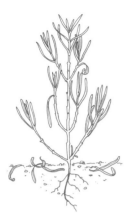

Root rot, which is caused by a fungus, occurs in overly wet soil.

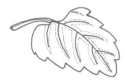

Viral infections cause plants to streak, discolor, and grow misshapen leaves.

Root rot can kill your plants before you know it has happened. Suspect root rot if your herb plants inexplicably lose leaves, turn brown, and die. It is caused by a fungus that is encouraged by overly wet conditions. When dug up, the roots of the plant will be brown-black and rotted. Prevent root rot by providing good drainage for your herbs, whether they are in beds or containers. Do not overwater herbs — let the soil dry out between waterings, if possible. Most herbs like to be a bit on the "dry" side. The herbs that are most susceptible to root rot are lavender, rosemary, sage, and thyme.

Viruses will cause your leaves to have yellow patches or streaks; they may become misshapen. Insects spread viruses, so controlling them will help prevent viruses on your herbs. Infected plants should be destroyed, not composted.

Garden tools can carry diseases from plant to plant. Any garden tools that come into contact with infected plants must be cleaned with rubbing alcohol or a 10 percent bleach solution and allowed to dry before they touch other plants.

Treating Plant Diseases

Should disease strike your herb plants, remove and destroy all of those affected. Do not put diseased plants on your compost pile; the diseases can be carried over wherever you apply the compost. If disease strikes your container-grown herbs, destroy the plant and the soil and thoroughly clean the container with a 10 percent bleach solution (1 part bleach to 9 parts water) before using it again. Do not plant the same variety of herb in a spot where disease has struck. Plant a different herb and wait 2 to 3 years before replacing it with the original variety.

When shopping for herb plants, check with your nurseries for any varieties resistant to commonly occurring diseases. If your gardens tend to harbor diseases, then it might be worth your money to buy the disease-resistant varieties.

USING A SPRAYER

A sprayer can be as small as a handheld bottle or as large as a tank that must be pulled on a trailer by another vehicle. Use the size that fits your needs. Mix substances only when you need them, and follow the label directions. Thoroughly clean the spray equipment after each use, allowing it to dry out between uses.

It is best to pick a quiet day to use a sprayer, to prevent the spray from drifting onto other plants. Do not spray in early-morning hours, when honeybees and other beneficial insects are actively foraging; helpful insects can be harmed by spraying, too. Despite the "nontoxic" label on these insecticides, many do not differentiate between good and bad insects.

CHAPTER 9

Harvesting and Storing Your Herbs

ou've gone to all of the trouble to plant the herbs. They've been growing and doing well. Now what do you do with them next? When harvested, preserved, and stored properly, your herbs will be in the best possible condition for year-round use. Follow the guidelines given here to harvest, preserve, and store your herbs for optimum quality.

HERBAL HARVEST

The best time to harvest depends on what part of the plant you want to use. If you are harvesting the plant for its leaves and/or stems, you'd ideally harvest it before it flowers. Flowering requires quite a bit of energy and takes away from the strength of the plant's essential oils. To harvest flowers, remove them from the plant just as they are opening. Seeds should be harvested when they are dry and starting to fall from the plant. Roots are best harvested in fall, after the plant has grown throughout the season.

Sharp Instruments Required

Use very clean, sharp scissors or hand pruners for harvesting. Pinching and pulling on leaves, flowers, and stems can crush plant parts and cause damage. Pulling and tugging can dislodge the plant from the soil, too.

Time of Day

Morning is the best time of day to reap your herbal harvest. Herbs, with the exception of calendula, are at their best in the morning. Wait until the dew has dried. If morning is not a good time to harvest for you, do it when you have the time.

Gathering Annuals, Biennials, and Perennials

The age of your herb plants will determine how much that you can harvest from them without hindering their growth. Young plants can tolerate only light harvests. For young annuals like dill, and biennials such as parsley in their first year, harvest small amounts of the herbs at the beginning of the growing season. As the weeks pass and the herbs grow, you can harvest up to one-third of their stems and foliage at a time.

Perennials harvested for their foliage include catnip, fennel, feverfew, lemon balm, peppermint, rosemary, sage, sweet marjoram, thyme, and yarrow. Ideally, you'll cut them for harvest before they bloom. Harvest newly planted perennials very lightly until they are well established and showing vigorous growth. Then you may harvest one-third of the plant at a time.

For annual flowering herbs such as calendula and German chamomile, biennial flowering herbs like red clover, and the perennial flowering herb yarrow, you can harvest the flowers as they open. You will have to be diligent and do this on a daily or semidaily basis, for the flowers won't all be in bloom at once. As the season progresses, the annuals will grow and bloom more. I like to leave a few flowers of each annual plant to self-seed, so that I'll have a new crop next season. Lavender buds are an exception to the rule of harvesting flowers when they first open: Harvest lavender when the flowers are unopened buds.

Harvesting Seeds, Roots, and Rhizomes

Herbs harvested for their seeds include dill and fennel. Wait until the seeds dry and are falling from the plant. If you shake a seed head and seeds start to fall, it is time to harvest.

Plants harvested for their roots or rhizomes include echinacea, ginger, and valerian. Dig up these plants in fall as you would to divide them. (See page 171.) Remove one-third to one-half of the roots or rhizomes; replant the remainder of the plants. Wash the soil from the roots and rhizomes, spread them out, and dry them thoroughly.

Important Harvest Tips

Aloe leaves are harvested for their gel. They are best picked as needed so that the gel is as fresh as possible. Pick cayenne peppers when they are bright red. Cut them from the plant with the stem intact; pulling can break off a main stem or branch. Dig garlic in fall. Let the bulbs dry with the stems intact to prevent spoiling. For further information on the harvest of any of the herbs in this book, check the individual profiles found in Herbs to Know and Appreciate.

For all harvests, remember:

- Do not harvest any diseased plants for use.
- Do not harvest any herbs for use that have been exposed to herbicides or pesticides.
- Shake the harvested parts vigorously to evict any insects that may be hiding before bringing in your harvest.
- If plant parts that you want to harvest are dusty and/or dirty, spray them clean with water the day before you harvest. They will be dry and clean by the next day.
- When you prune or thin a plant, include the parts you remove as part of your herbal harvest.
- Harvest sparingly from young or newly established plants.

PRESERVING YOUR HARVEST

There are several ways to preserve herbs, ranging from simple methods that require little or no investment in equipment to more expensive ways. Drying is the primary method of preserving herbs, but I have outlined some other options as well.

Drying Herb Leaves

When harvesting your herb leaves, keep them on their stems. Use a string or rubber band to fasten the ends of the stems together into a bundle. Tie the bundle upside down and hang it in a dry place that is out of direct sunlight and heat. Check the leaves after a few days for dryness. When the leaves are crisp and crumbly, they are dry; take them down as soon as possible or they will reabsorb moisture from the air. Using your fingers, strip the leaves from the stems and store them in a tightly closed glass container, away from heat and light.

A slow cooker can also dry herb leaves. Cut the herb stems into a size that will fit into the appliance. Fill it with herbs to about one-third to one-half full. Turn it to its lowest setting and, with the lid off, let the herbs dry. Gently turn the herbs occasionally to enhance the drying process. When the leaves are crisp and crumbly, they are dry. Using your fingers, strip them from the stems and store them in a tightly closed glass container, away from heat and light.

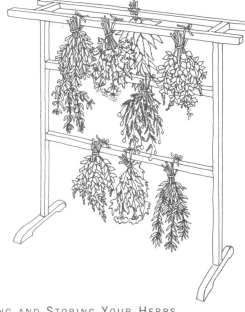

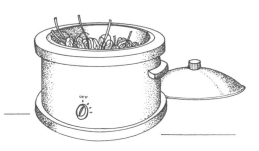

Tie bundles of herbs together and hang them upside down to dry (left). A slow cooker can be used to dry herb leaves and flowers (above).

Using a food dehydrator is another way to dry herbs. Cut the herbs to fit into the dehydrator and follow the manufacturer's instructions. After drying, use your fingers to strip the leaves from the stem. Store your dried herbs in a tightly closed glass container, away from heat and light.

Drying Herb Flowers

Flowers are much more delicate than leaves and should be dried gently. After picking the flowers, place them in a single layer on a drying rack. (This can be purchased or made from a raised wooden frame over which you've stretched cheesecloth or nylon net. A clean metal window screen laid flat could also be used. Place the rack in a dry place away from direct sunlight. Let flowers sit there until they are thoroughly dry. The amount of drying time varies according to the humidity in the air, but it generally takes one to two weeks. Store them in a tightly closed glass container, away from heat and light.

You can also dry flowers with the slow-cooker method I described above. It will not take flowers as long to dry as leaves, so keep a close eye on them. Turn the flowers every 15 to 30 minutes during the drying process.

Commercial dehydrators can also be used to dry herb flowers. Place the flowers in a single layer in the dehydrator, and follow the instructions from your manufacturer. Store the dried flowers in a tightly closed glass container in a cool, dark place.

Lavender is harvested and dried differently. Cut the herb's stems long enough to tie into bundles to dry. If the lavender buds are all you need, strip them from the stems after they are dry and store. Or, you can use a commercial dehydrator to dry lavender.

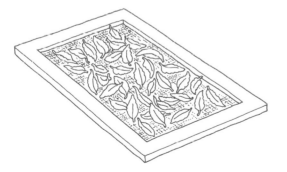

Spread herb leaves or flowers in a single layer on a wooden drying rack or clean window screen.

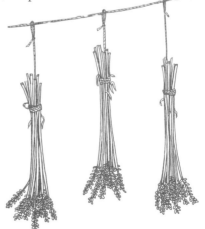

Lavender is best when air-dried in long-stemmed bundles.

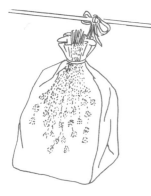

Seeds will fall off the plant when dry. To contain them, place herb bundles inside a paper bag, punch a few holes into the top, and tie shut.

Drying Herb Seeds

Herb seeds are dry when they are falling from the plant. To gather the drying seeds of dill or fennel, cut the seed heads from the plants leaving an approximately 8-inch-long stem on each. Bundle up the stems with string or a rubber band. Place the seed heads upside down in a paper bag and tie the bag opening around the stems with a string. Hang the bag in a dry place out of direct sunlight. As the seeds dry, they will fall into the bag. After most of the seeds have fallen, remove the bag and strip any remaining seeds off the seed heads with your fingers. Transfer the seeds from the bag to a glass container. Store in a cool, dark place.

Drying Herb Roots

After cleaning and washing, cut up roots into smaller (about ½-inch) pieces. Dry them in a commercial dehydrator following the manufacturer's directions. Store the dried root pieces as you would any herb, in a tightly closed glass container and away from heat and light.

Another drying technique for roots is the slow-cooker method. (See page 194.) You can use your oven, too. Place the root pieces in a single layer on a tray or cookie sheet. Turn your oven to its lowest setting and put the tray or sheet inside, leaving the door open an inch or two. The roots are ready when they feel dry and hard (this will take several hours). Look for them to shrink somewhat.

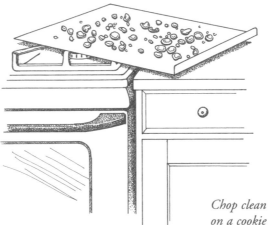

Chop clean herb roots and dry them on a cookie sheet in the oven.

Microwave?

Because of the method's ease and quickness, some books and herb growers swear by drying herbs in the microwave oven. I don't recommend it, however, because it is quite difficult to judge the proper amount of time to dry herbs in a microwave. With herbs dried in the microwave, there is a very fine line between dry and burned.

Freezing Herbs

Frozen feverfew leaves are almost as good fresh, and you can use them year-round. Pick the clean, dry leaves individually before the plant is in bloom and stack them up. Place the stacked leaves in a resealable plastic bag, label with the herb name and date, and place in the freezer for future use. When you want to use a feverfew leaf, just remove one from the bag then reseal and replace the bag in the freezer.

Cayenne peppers and parsley can each be chopped with a little water then placed in ice cube trays. After freezing, transfer the cubes to a resealable plastic bag. Label the bag with the name and date, then store in the freezer. When you want to use either herb, take out as many cubes out as you need.

Ginger rhizomes can be stored easily in the freezer, too. Place the clean and dry rhizome in a resealable plastic bag, label with the name and date, and freeze. Cut or grate the amount of the rhizome that you need directly from the freezer, then replace what you haven't used.

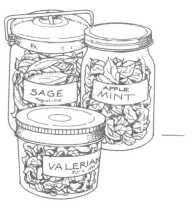

Other herbs discussed in this book do not freeze well; freezing affects their color and texture. When thawed, the herbs are often dark and mushy. I do not recommend this process for any herbs other than feverfew, cayenne pepper, parsley, and ginger.

Other methods of herb preservation involve extracting the active ingredients of the herb and combining it with another substance. Herbal infused oils and tinctures are examples of these extraction methods. See pages 12–14 for instructions.

Always store herbs in clear, covered, and labeled bottles and jars.

Storage of Dried Herbs

Heat and sunlight are the enemies of the active ingredients in dried herbs; both will cause the herbs to lose their potency. Therefore, it is important to expose drying herbs to heat only long enough to dry them, then store immediately.

Glass containers with snug-fitting lids are the best storage containers for dried herbs. Dark-colored glass containers are even better, but they're not always easy to find. Clean, empty food jars and canning jars can be used.

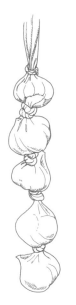

Twist garlic bulbs into a length of old nylon stocking, and tie knots between each bulb.

Avoid crumbling dried herbs completely before storing; essential oils are more likely to stay intact in larger pieces. Instead, crumble the herbs immediately prior to use. You can grind roots into finer pieces, if desired, with an electric coffee grinder just before use.

Place all preserved herbs in individual jars. Label each jar with the name of the herb and the date. Store the jars out of direct sunlight and away from intense heat. The first week after you stored the herbs, check them closely. If there is any sign of moisture condensation on the inside of the jar, the herbs have not been properly dried and must be discarded, as this moisture can cause the herbs to mold. If there is any sign of mold, you must discard the herbs and start over.

A drastic fading of the color of the dried herbs compared to when they were first stored also indicates a loss of potency. Discard the herbs if they fade in this way, and consider changing the area where you store them. Your original storage area is probably receiving too much heat and light.

Dried herb leaves and flowers will remain useful for up to 2 years, and roots will last from 2 to 3 years when stored properly. If you dry and store herbs throughout your growing season, this storage time will keep you in herbs all through the winter months, until the next growing and harvesting season.

Garlic: The Exception

Garlic bulbs need to be stored in a cool, dry, well-ventilated place. Recycled net bags provide appropriate storage, as do old clean nylon stockings. After you put each garlic bulb in the stocking, tie a knot above it, then add another garlic bulb and tie another knot. Continue until all of your garlic is stored. When you want to use some, cut the first bulb out of the stocking. Store the part of the bulb that you don't use in a small crock with ventilation holes. These are made specifically for garlic storage and work quite well.

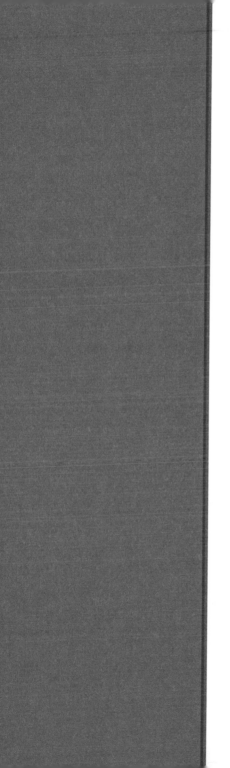

CHAPTER 10

Gathering the Wild Things

When I became interested in herbs, one of the facts that I learned is that useful plants are everywhere. Many plants that I once scorned and pulled from my garden for the weeds that they were have taken on a new status in my eyes. I have even been known to stop along a roadside while biking to inspect a plant and perhaps take cuttings of it home for further study, a habit that my son finds embarrassing when he is with me. (Either he thinks I am trespassing, or he is concerned one of his friends might see me employed in this strange task!)

I have actually incorporated some of these plants into the meals I cook, enticed by the vitamins and minerals they contain. My frugal nature is satisfied by these plants. They are useful, healthful, and plentiful without having to be cultivated.

Instead of cursing the presence of these plants and trying to rid them from your yard and garden, learn about their usefulness and live in harmony with them. They can give you and your family some nutritional and medicinal benefits. A bonus is that you may find your attitude about wild plants changing as you use them. Besides, isn't it a positive step in your life to replace an attitude of contempt with one of respect?

There are regional differences in the types of wild plants available. Check out a good guidebook on wild plants to see what grows near you. It is also a good idea to work with someone knowledgeable about useful wild plants in your area.

A ROYAL DECREE FOR HERBALISTS

"Be it ordained, established, and enacted by Authority of this present Parliament, that at all Time from henceforth it shall be lawful to every Person being the King's subject having Knowledge and Experience of the Nature of Herbs, Roots and Waters, or of the Operation of the same . . . within any part of the Realm of England or within any other under the King's Dominions, to practice, use, and minister in and to any . . ."

—Herbalists Charter of Henry VIII

HARVESTING DOS AND DON'TS

Some rules to follow when you are looking for wild plants to harvest include these:

- Do ask permission to hunt for plants on land that belongs to someone besides you. It is common courtesy to do so, and considered trespassing if you don't.
- Do be absolutely sure that you are harvesting the right plant. Correct identification is essential, because some plants are quite poisonous. Take a good plant identification book along with you, preferably one with color photographs, and/or go with someone who has a working knowledge of wild plants.
- Don't harvest and use any plant that has been exposed to potentially harmful chemicals. You should be particularly aware of this when you're hunting for plants in unfamiliar territory, but it's true of plants harvested from your yard as well; if you treat your lawn with herbicides and pesticides, you should not be eating any plants gathered from it.
- Don't harvest all of the plants in one area. Leave some to reproduce and for future use.
- Don't pick plants that are endangered. The organization United Plant Savers can give you information on endangered plants. (See Resources.)

Harvesting at a High Price

The popularity of using herbs medicinally, the destruction of natural habitat, and the high prices charged for wild-gathered herbs are taking a toll on wild plant populations. A few of the plants included on United Plant Savers' "At Risk" list are American ginseng, echinacea, goldenseal, and slippery elm. Without judicious harvesting practices and preservation programs, many of our most useful wild plants will disappear.

What is being done to help? United Plant Savers is establishing botanical sanctuaries, and has initiated a public education program. Frontier Natural Products Co-op has begun a program of growing at-risk herbs. Their successful Goldenseal Project has allowed them to cultivate goldenseal for sale to customers.

For more information on many endangered herbs, contact United Plant Savers (see Resources).

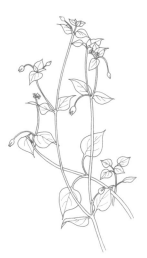

Chickweed (Stellaria media)

Either overlooked or much maligned, this little plant has several potential uses. I always take a sample of chickweed to classes to let people see in a new light a plant usually eliminated from the garden.

Named *Stellaria* because of its white starlike flowers, it is commonly seen grown in cultivated ground and is low growing. The plant's properties include nutritive, astringent, demulcent, and vulnerary.

Food and Medicinal Uses

The nutritional value of chickweed is impressive. It contains vitamins A, B, C, and D, as well as phosphorus, zinc, and calcium. I always sprinkle a few of the little leaves in green salads from the garden. The taste is subtle and adds many nutrients to the mix.

An infusion of chickweed applied externally can help to relieve the itching of irritating skin conditions. Internally, the infusion can be taken for relief from the discomfort of urinary tract infections. It is also thought to help relieve the mucus buildup of colds and bronchitis.

I made a chickweed infusion for my son when he had chicken pox. Add ½ cup fresh or ¼ cup dried chickweed to 2 cups water. Simmer for 15 minutes, then strain. Allow the infusion to cool before applying as a lotion to itchy areas of skin. For an internal chickweed infusion, use 1 tablespoon fresh or 2 teaspoons dried to 1 cup boiling water. Let steep for 10 minutes, strain, and sip. Do not drink more than 1 cup of this infusion a day.

An infused oil or ointment made with chickweed can be applied to itchy skin conditions. When applied to minor wounds or splinters embedded in the skin, it can help to draw out the foreign body of the splinter and any infections present.

As with any substance, moderation is in order with chickweed. Eating excessive amounts of it, or drinking too much of its infusion, can possibly cause the breakdown of red blood cells. This is due to the herb's high content of a substance called saponin.

MAKING CHICKWEED OINTMENT

Keep a jar of this in your medicine chest for use in drawing out splinters or healing minor cuts and scrapes.

Follow the instructions for infused oil on page 12, but use dried chickweed for the herb. Melt together 4½ tablespoons chickweed-infused oil and 2 tablespoons beeswax in a heatproof container over boiling water. Remove from heat. Add 800 IU vitamin E as a preservative. Store in a low, widemouthed jar.

Chicory *(Cichorium intybus)*

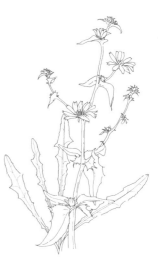

Chicory has been cultivated for thousands of years. Egyptian records detail its growth and use there five thousand years ago. It made a popular drink in England; even Queen Elizabeth I drank chicory broth. The plant was naturalized in North America. Thomas Jefferson planted chicory seeds from Italy in his Monticello gardens.

I first became aware of chicory while driving down the road one summertime. There they grew along the roadside, tall plants with shaggy sky blue flowers. I gathered some seeds and planted my own patch. Now I only have to step outside my door to enjoy the blooms. I have a bonus, too: Goldfinches love the seeds and will perch among the spent blooms to feast. What a sight to see the vibrant blue and yellow together!

Food and Medicinal Uses

Chicory is another wild plant that is a powerhouse of nutrients. The green leaves are high in vitamin A, calcium, and potassium, as well as containing phosphorus, iron, and vitamins C and B. The leaves' properties include stomachic, tonic, cholagogue, diuretic, and laxative.

The deep taproot grows best in deeply worked soil, but will certainly grow in poor, heavy clay soils as well. Studies have shown the root to have antibacterial and anti-inflammatory properties. An infusion of the root stimulates bile secretion and tones an upset stomach. The fresh root contains inulin, a concentrated source of dietary fiber that is safe for diabetics. Studies are currently being done on the effect of chicory root on the heart. Chicory flower petals are used in one of the Bach Flower Remedies (remedies formulated from plants) to help people who are overpossessive and demanding of attention overcome these traits.

Roasted chicory roots will provide you with a coffee substitute that is caffeine-free; you can also add the roots to your coffee to smooth its taste. The petals of the chicory flower are edible and can be sprinkled fresh on salads. Eat the leaves fresh — the young ones are more tender and less bitter than the older.

Growing Chicory

Cultivated chicory varieties include radicchio and endive; you can purchase seeds through many seed companies. To obtain seeds of the wild variety, gather them from a plant found in the wild. Wild chicory will bloom continuously for several weeks and requires little care. Be aware that chicory self-seeds with abandon and, once established, is difficult to move due to its deep taproot; plant it somewhere so that it can spread.

> ## ROASTED CHICORY ROOT
>
> To roast chicory roots, clean them well. Cut them into ¼- to ½-inch slices and place on an ungreased baking sheet. Roast in 200°F (93°C) oven until the root pieces are very dry and brown in color. Cool thoroughly and store in a tightly closed glass container. Roasted roots can be ground and blended with coffee or drunk on their own as a coffee substitute.

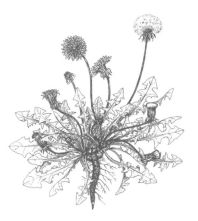

Dandelion *(Taraxacum officinale)*

This is one of the most maligned herbs in our country; you can scarcely pick up any gardening literature without seeing ads for herbicides that get rid of dandelions.

This negative attitude toward dandelions was not shared by our ancestors. The plant was valued as a useful medicinal as early as the 10th century, and the regard continued for several hundred more years. The herb's worth was great enough that dandelion seeds were brought to North America by early European settlers.

Food and Medicinal Uses

All parts of the dandelion except the stem are edible. The root contains vitamin C and inulin. The roots are thought to filter toxins and wastes from the bloodstream. Ingesting them also stimulates bile flow; for this reason, they have been used to treat liver disorders. You can roast and grind them to use as a coffee substitute, too.

The jagged edges of the green leaves give the plant its common name, which is derived from the French *dent de lion,* meaning "lion's tooth." The leaves contain iron, potassium, calcium, and vitamins A, B, C, and D. In fact, there is more calcium in dandelion leaves than in an equivalent amount of milk! Dandelion greens are more nutritious than spinach; they also have diuretic and laxative effects.

The beautiful shaggy yellow flowers give some bright color to your lawn sooner than most cultivated varieties of flowers. The flower buds contain the nutrient lecithin and are edible. The flowers are the main ingredient in dandelion wine.

Not Just for Food and Medicine!

Last but not least, the round seed heads give children the pleasant pastime of making wishes and blowing the seeds off. When our son was quite young, he would hit the seed heads with a stick. There he would stand in a cloud of dandelion seeds and watch them fly or float away. Don't scold children for scattering the seeds; use this as a learning opportunity. And next spring, look at the dandelions in your yard with more respect.

Dandelion Cooking Hints

You can eat dandelion leaves fresh or cooked when they are young and tender. To rid them of some of their bitter taste, briefly blanch them in boiling water, remove and rinse in cool water, then prepare them as you have planned. To cook the flower buds, soak them for an hour or two in salted water, drain thoroughly, then sauté in butter or margarine. You can also bread and fry them.

DANDELION CAUTIONS

The milky white latex in the stems has been known to cause children to become ill when they suck on the stems.

Don't ingest any parts of the dandelion plant if you experience bile duct problems or have a history of gall stones.

Goldenrod *(Solidago* spp.)

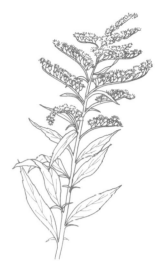

This spectacular-looking plant has an undeserved reputation. Its pollen has been blamed for allergy and hay fever problems for years. The fact is that goldenrod pollen is sticky and doesn't float in the air to irritate people who are susceptible. (The more likely culprit for irritation is ragweed pollen.)

Goldenrod has been used for centuries medicinally. In the Middle Ages, Arabs promoted the herb for its anti-inflammatory, expectorant, vulnerary, astringent, and weak diuretic properties. Chinese herbalists also used it. Native Americans as well as Europeans have long used it. After the Boston Tea Party, colonists in North America drank a tea of the leaves to replace the tea that they so enjoyed but refused to drink.

Medicinal Uses

The plant's essential oil has antiseptic and expectorant properties. One of the constituents of this essential oil is borneol, an ingredient frequently found in natural topical decongestant preparations.

A wide variety of ailments has been treated with an infusion of goldenrod leaves. Europeans widely use the infusion to treat respiratory problems such as colds and bronchitis. When drunk, the infusion is also agreeable to an upset stomach. An infusion made from the blossoms has been regarded as a general tonic, and used as a headache remedy.

The leaves are used in salves that can be applied to wounds and insect bites.

Due to its diuretic properties, goldenrod is used in Europe to treat urinary tract inflammation. If you have a pre-existing kidney disease or a chronic kidney disorder, consult your health-care provider about taking goldenrod. Take along literature that describes the action of goldenrod; herbs and their actions are not well known to many health-care providers.

Growing Goldenrod

Goldenrod is regarded as a beautiful addition to flower and herb gardens in Europe. I am of the opinion that it should be included in North American gardens as well. It provides wonderful golden yellow color in late summer and fall when many plants have finished blooming. Its height (3–4 feet) makes it a beautiful addition to the back of your flower and herb beds. It is best propagated by root divisions.

Goldenrod is drought tolerant and will grow best in poor soils. It is relatively pest-free. The humidity of summer can cause the leaves to have some powdery mildew.

USING GOLDENROD INFUSION

This can be made with either leaves or flowers. Do not drink more than 1½ cups of infusion a day, and do not drink the infusion if you are allergic to goldenrod.

Add 1 to 2 teaspoons of the dried herb to 1 cup water. Bring the mixture to a boil, then remove it from the heat and let it stand, covered, for 2 to 5 minutes. Strain and drink.

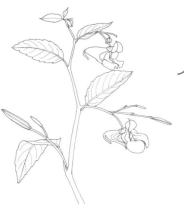

Jewelweed *(Impatiens capensis)*

Last summer I found myself wading through waist-high grasses and weeds in our front field on an unplanned errand. The undergrowth was thick with poison ivy and my legs were bare. After my expedition, I found a lush patch of jewelweed. I broke off several of the plants, crushed them in my hand, and rubbed them on my poison-ivy-exposed legs. I waited a couple of days to see if I broke out in the rash typical of poison ivy exposure. It didn't happen. Once again, herbs helped me out.

Jewelweed is a beautiful plant of the impatiens family. Its name comes from either its beautiful little red-orange or yellow flowers, or the glistening drops of moisture that bead up on its leaves after a rain or heavy dew. It likes damp places and partial shade. After flowering, the plant self-seeds. Nature frequently provides us with an immediate treatment for poison ivy exposure since jewelweed can often be found growing near poison ivy patches. Teach your children to recognize and avoid poison ivy. Likewise, teach them how to recognize and use jewelweed.

Medicinal Uses

Jewelweed plants can easily be used directly on skin exposed to poison ivy. Just pick a fresh plant, crush it in your hand, and rub it on affected areas. An active ingredient in jewelweed has been shown in studies to help relieve the itch of hives when topically applied. I am hopeful that more research will be done concerning that use.

JEWELWEED INFUSION

To relieve the itch of poison ivy rash (or to apply to skin exposed to poison ivy to help prevent a reaction), try this externally applied infusion. Do not make a jewelweed tincture: When mixed with alcohol and applied topically, jewelweed can cause severe skin reactions.

For the infusion, use 1 part jewelweed to 20 parts distilled water. Strain the plant from the infusion and freeze the liquid in an ice cube tray. These cubes can be stored in a labeled resealable plastic bag; the infusion liquid can also be refrigerated for a week.

Lamb's-Quarter *(Chenopodium album)*

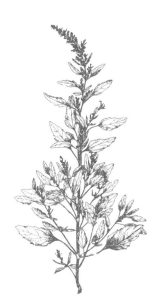

I just can't leave this common weed out of my wild herbs list. It is a tasty and nutritious addition to meals. It grows readily just about anywhere that it drops seeds, and is tolerant of many soil and growing conditions. Last spring I wrote an article about eating lamb's-quarter and still receive surprised comments about it.

Nutritional and Medicinal Uses

This weed is high in vitamin A, and contains vitamin C, iron, and calcium. Lamb's-quarter belongs in the same family as beets and Swiss chard. The taste of the leaves is comparable with that of spinach. Take advantage of its versatility and harvest the leaves to eat cooked or fresh sprinkled in a salad.

Unlike some wild plants, the flavor of lamb's-quarter leaves is mild. The small brown seeds are also considered palatable; they can be ground and used in place of half the flour in a recipe, or cooked and eaten as hot cereal. What a lot to offer from a scorned plant!

Lamb's-Quarter with Herbs

When the spinach in your garden is long gone, harvest the leaves of lamb's-quarter and serve this dish instead. Other flavorful herbs can be substituted for the garlic or garlic chives.

- 3 cups lamb's-quarter leaves, washed with the stems removed
- ½ cup chopped fresh herbs of your choice (I like to add garlic chives or peeled, chopped garlic cloves)
- 1 teaspoon vegetable oil
- Salt and pepper to taste

Sauté the lamb's-quarter and herbs in the oil just until the leaves start to wilt. Add salt and pepper to taste and serve.

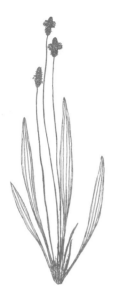

Plantain *(Plantago major, P. lanceolata)*

This common plant can be found almost anywhere you look. In Europe plantain was a useful medicinal for ancient European and Germanic tribes. Anglo-Saxons considered it an important healing herb; it was included as one of their nine sacred herbs. After plantain was brought to North America by European settlers, the Natives came to call it "white man's footprint" because it grew wherever the white man lived.

Food and Medicinal Uses

Two parts of plantain are considered useful. The leaves have relaxing, astringent, antispasmodic, refrigerant, and expectorant properties. They are also tonic to mucous membranes and are known to reduce phlegm. When crushed and placed on skin injuries, irritations, or insect stings, the leaves can provide relief and promote healing. An infusion of the leaves can aid in relieving coughs and can be used to soothe an irritated stomach.

The seed husks are included in many commercial bulk laxative products. The husks have cells that contain mucilage, which is not digested or absorbed in the intestines. These cells swell to a large size when they come into contact with water, so you must drink large amounts of water when taking the seed husks for them to be effective as a bulk laxative. An additional positive effect is that mucilage in your diet is thought to help lower cholesterol levels.

Plantain leaves are most palatable when they are young and small. The older leaves are too tough to be enjoyed in salads. Plantain seeds and their husks are quite small. Harvesting the seeds to obtain the husks is quite impractical and labor intensive, so it is a better idea to buy commercial bulk laxative products if this is what you need.

EAT YOUR PLANTAIN

The narrow-leafed variety of plantain *(P. lanceolata)* is thought to be more tender than the broad-leafed variety *(P. major)*, although I have not noticed a great difference between the two. The uncooked young tender leaves of either variety are best when added to mixed-green spring salads. The young leaves can also be sautéed in butter or olive oil and seasoned with salt, pepper, and herbs or your choice. You may cook the leaves alone or try them in combination with other wild greens such as dandelion, chicory, or lamb's-quarter. The older plantain leaves are tough and fibrous, and I do not recommend trying to eat them — either cooked or uncooked.

Purslane *(Portulaca oleracea)*

This is another plant that seems to appear in my gardens without being deliberately planted. It is low growing with succulent leaves and stems. It commonly is found growing in light and rich cultivated soil.

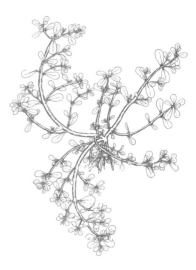

Nutritional and Medicinal Uses

The tangy flavor of young purslane leaves and stems makes them tasty additions to any salad, and the amount of nutrients they contain will persuade you to include them the next time you make a salad. Purslane contains vitamins A, C, D, and K, as well as calcium, magnesium, phosphorus, potassium, and iron. It is important to note that purslane also has high levels of the beneficial omega-3 fatty acids, which can affect cholesterol levels and reduce the risk of blood clots and heart attack.

Purslane is made up mostly of water — over 90 percent, by some accounts. This makes it an appropriate "diet" food. If you want a low-calorie, nutritious green, purslane is a good choice.

Spring Greens Salad

Welcome the arrival of longer days and renewed growing with this vitamin-packed mixture. Use any combination of wild herbs, according to your tastes and what you find growing.

- 6 cups new lettuce
- 2 cups mixed new dandelion leaves, chicory leaves, chickweed leaves, lamb's-quarter leaves, and purslane stems and leaves

Tear the lettuce and other leaves into bite-size pieces. Toss and serve with an herbal-infused vinegar and oil dressing.

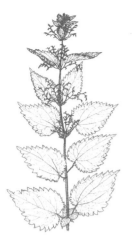

Stinging Nettle *(Urtica dioica)*

This plant presents an unfriendly face to the world with its uncomfortable stinging hairs. It takes an open mind to look past this stinging to see its potential uses. Nettles are said to grow in rich, fertile soil. The seeds of stinging nettle can be purchased for planting but I have never had the nerve to plant them in my gardens!

In past cultures, stinging nettle was seen in a much more positive light. It was considered a sacred plant in Scandinavia. The seeds were brought to England by the Romans. They rubbed the plants on their bodies to help keep themselves warm, using the stinging sensation to their advantage.

Nutritional and Medicinal Uses

In past and present times stinging nettle has been used to treat bronchitis and asthma, and to provide hay-fever relief. Fresh stinging-nettle plants have been applied to arthritic joints to help provide pain relief, an action that is not proved in scientific research, but well known as a folk cure. An infusion of nettle tea is antibacterial. This makes it a logical choice to use as a mouthwash.

The herb contains a high amount of iron and, when eaten once a week, will benefit the body. When drunk in an infusion it is said to strengthen and support the body as well as purify the blood. Other nutrients contained in stinging nettles include calcium, magnesium, silicon, and boron. The latter is a significant mineral to include in your diet, since it helps bones retain calcium.

To prepare nettles for food, wear gloves and collect the plants when they are young. Chop them up and sauté in a small amount of oil with onions and garlic. Cooking the nettles removes the sting from them. Do not eat nettles more than once a week.

MAKING NETTLE INFUSION

Add 1 to 2 teaspoons of dried nettles (the process of drying takes the sting out of them) to 1 cup of boiling water. Infuse for 10 to 15 minutes, then strain the herb from the infusion. Do not drink more than 2 cups of infusion a day.

Glossary

GARDENING TERMS

Aerial. The part of a plant that grows above the ground.

Annual. A plant that grows, blooms, produces seeds, and dies in one growing season.

Biennial. A plant that grows, flowers, produces seeds, and dies in a 2-year period.

Cells or cell packs. Containers manufactured with a given number of sections per piece for planting in a group.

Chlorophyll. The green color in plants that is responsible for the absorption of light.

Climate. The average annual weather conditions for a given area, including temperature, winds, and precipitation.

Compost. Organic material formed from the decomposed parts of discarded plant materials of various kinds. Used as a soil additive or mulch.

Deadheading. Removing flowers or flower heads past their prime.

Division. A way to propagate plants by dividing into pieces.

Dormancy. The slowing of growth and other activities of a plant, usually during cold-weather months.

Drainage. The passage of excess water through the soil.

Germination. The changes that take place in a seed when it begins to grow and develop into a plant.

Green up. The new green growth of plants after a period of rest or dormancy. Usually seen in the spring in areas that have cold winters.

Growing zone. Parts of continents are divided into zones, determined by average annual minimum temperatures. These are also known as Hardiness Zones.

Insecticide. A natural or synthetic substance used to kill and/or control insects. (*See* Pesticide.)

Layering. A method of propagation in which a shoot is encouraged to grow roots.

Mulch. A natural or man-made material placed on the ground to suppress weeds, conserve moisture, and moderate soil temperature.

Node. A "joint" on the stem of the plant. Stems, leaves, flowers, and, in some cases, roots can arise from nodes.

Organic gardening. Growing plants without the use of synthetic or nonorganic materials.

Overwinter. The ability of plants to survive winter and grow the next year.

Perennial. A plant whose life span is at least three seasons.

Pesticide. A natural or synthetic substance used to kill and/or control insects. (*See* Insecticide.)

Propagation. The act of increasing the number of plants that you have by a variety of methods.

Rhizome. A plant stem that grows underground and stores food. Shoots grow along the rhizome and become the aerial part of the plant.

Rootball. The roots and accompanying soil or potting mix that is present when a plant is either removed from a container or the ground.

Runner. A horizontally spreading stem that runs above ground and forms roots on nodes of the stem.

Self-seed. In plants, to drop fertile seeds around the mother plant.

Semievergreen. Plants that retain a small part of their leaves for more than one season.

Soil. The upper layer of earth where plants can grow.

Stem cutting. A portion of the stem of a plant that is cut off to be used for propagation.

Stratification. The process of storing seeds in cool conditions to promote germination by breaking dormancy.

Succulent. A plant with thick, fleshy leaves that are made expressly to store water.

Taproot. The primary downward-growing root of a plant.

Tender perennial. A frost-tender plant whose life span is at least three seasons given the appropriate temperatures.

Topsoil. The uppermost layer of the soil.

Umbel. A group of small flowers blooming from a number of similar sized flower stalks that grow on a single stem. These flowers form a flat top.

Vermiculite. A lightweight mineral that is added to soil or potting mix to enhance drainage. It is also useful when stratifying seeds.

Viable. Capable of growing or developing.

MEDICAL TERMS

Analgesic. A substance that relieves pain.

Antibacterial. A substance that works to inhibit the growth of bacteria.

Antidepressant. A substance that relieves depression.

Antiemetic. A substance that relieves vomiting or nausea.

Antifungal. A substance that has the ability to inhibit the growth of fungi.

Antihidrotic. A substance that inhibits sweating.

Anti-inflammatory. A substance that counteracts inflammation.

Antimicrobial. A substance that inhibits the growth of microorganisms.

Antioxidant. A substance that blocks or slows oxidation, which produces free radicals — potentially destructive compounds that can cause cell damage.

Antiseptic. A substance that prevents the growth of microorganisms.

Antispasmodic. A substance that prevents or relieves spasms or cramps.

Antiviral. A substance that works against viruses.

Aromatic. Having a strong smell that can potentially have therapeutic use.

Astringent. A substance that increases the tone of tissues.

Ayurvedic. Pertaining to Ayurveda, a science of healing that originated in India.

Carminative. A substance that stimulates the expulsion of gas from the gastrointestinal tract.

Cathartic. Having a strong laxative effect.

Cholagogue. A substance that promotes the flow of bile.

Counterirritant. A substance that, when applied locally, produces skin-surface redness that reduces inflammation in adjacent tissues. (*See* Rubefacient.)

Decoction. A liquid in which an herb has been simmered in order to extract its active properties. This method is used for roots and bark.

Demulcent. A substance that softens and soothes irritation of mucous membranes.

Diaphoretic. A substance that promotes perspiration.

Digestive. A substance that aids in digestion.

Diuretic. A substance that expels water, thus increasing the flow of urine.

Dyspepsia. Indigestion, or difficulty in digesting.

Eczema. An inflammatory skin condition.

Emmenagogue. A substance that promotes menstruation.

Emollient. A topical substance applied to soften and smooth the skin.

Essential oil. The concentrated oil found in herbs that contain their active ingredients. The oil often has a distinctive, strong aroma.

Expectorant. A substance that promotes the elimination of mucus from the respiratory tract.

Free radicals. Unstable compounds that can take oxygen from healthy cells, causing them damage and possibly destroying them.

Galactogogue. A substance that promotes the flow of breast milk in a nursing mother.

Hemostatic. A substance that stops bleeding.

Hypnotic. A substance that has the ability to induce sleep.

Hypotensive. A substance that lowers blood pressure.

Infused oil. Oil that has had herbs introduced to it in order to transfer the properties of the herbs into the oil.

Internal cleanser. A substance which, when taken internally, will aid in removing potentially harmful agents from the body.

Lymphatic. A substance that can stimulate and cleanse the lymphatic system.

Nervine. A substance that tones the nervous system.

Property. A quality or trait that belongs to a particular herb.

Relaxant. A substance that promotes relaxation.

Rubefacient. A substance applied locally to stimulate and increase blood flow to the skin's surface.

Salve. A substance that can be spread on the skin, made by combining an oil with an emulsifier such as beeswax, to achieve a stiff consistency.

Sedative. A substance that promotes a feeling of calm and quiet in the face of excitement or nervousness.

Spasmolytic. *See* Antispasmodic.

Stimulant. A substance that increases functional activity and energy in the body. This can be a temporary increase.

Stomachic. A substance that enhances stomach function.

Tea or infusion. Hot water in which herbs have been steeped in order to transfer the plant properties to the liquid. This method is used for more delicate plant parts such as leaves and flowers.

Tincture. A liquid made from alcohol or glycerine and water in which herbs have been steeped to extract their properties.

Tonic. A substance that increases tone, energy, and vigor in a specific part of the body.

Topical. Pertaining to the surface of the skin.

Ulceration. An open wound in the skin that involves underlying tissue.

Vasodilatory. A substance that causes the blood vessels to widen.

Visceral. Related to the internal organs of the body.

Vulnerary. A substance that promotes the healing of new cuts and wounds.

Recommended Reading

Balch, James F., M.D., and Phyllis A. Balch, C.N.C. *Prescription for Nutritional Healing.* Garden City Park, N.Y.: Avery Publishing Group, 1997.

Bradley, Fern Marshall, and Barbara W. Ellis. editors. *Rodale's All New Encyclopedia of Organic Gardening.* Emmaus, Penn.: Rodale Press, 1992.

Bremness, Leslie. *The Complete Book of Herbs.* New York: Dorling Kindersley, Inc., 1988.

Bubel, Nancy. *The New Seed Starters Handbook.* Emmaus, Penn.: Rodale Press, 1988.

Byers, Dorie. *Natural Body Basics — Making Your Own Cosmetics.* Bargersville, Ind.: Gooseberry Hill Publications Inc., 1996.

Clark, Ethne. *Herb Garden Design.* New York: MacMillan Company, 1995.

Denckla, Tanya. *The Organic Gardener's Home Reference.* Pownal, Vt.: Storey Communications, Inc., 1994.

Dodt, Colleen K. *Natural Baby Care.* Pownal, Vt.: Storey Communications, Inc., 1997.

Duke, James A., Ph.D., *The Green Pharmacy.* Emmaus, Penn.: Rodale Press, 1997.

Dunn, Teri. *100 Favorite Herbs.* New York: Metrobooks, 1998.

Foster, Steven, and James A. Duke, Ph.D. *A Field Guide to Medicinal Plants.* Boston: Houghton Mifflin Co., 1990.

Foster, Steven. *Echinacea — Nature's Immune Enhancer.* Rochester, Vt.: Healing Arts Press, 1991.

———. *Herbal Renaissance,* revised edition of *Herbal Bounty!* Salt Lake City: Gibbs-Smith Publisher, 1984.

Griggs, Barbara. *The Green Witch Herbal.* Rochester, Vt.: Healing Arts Press, 1994.

Jacobs, Betty E. M. *Growing and Using Herbs Successfully.* Pownal, Vt.: Storey Communications, Inc., 1981.

Kowalchik, Claire, and William H. Hylton, editors, *Rodale's Illustrated Encyclopedia of Herbs.* Emmaus, Penn.: Rodale Press, 1987.

Lima, Patrick. *The Harrowsmith Illustrated Book of Herbs.* Camden East, Ontario: Camden House Publishing Ltd., 1986.

McClure, Susan. *The Herb Gardener: A Guide for All Seasons.* Pownal, Vt.: Garden Way Publishing, 1996.

Mowrey, Daniel B., Ph.D. *The Scientific Validation of Herbal Medicine.* New Canaan, Conn.: Keats Publishing, Inc., 1986.

Ody, Penelope. *The Complete Medicinal Herbal.* New York: Dorling Kindersley, Inc., 1993.

———. *Home Herbal.* New York: Dorling Kindersley, Inc., 1995.

Reppert, Bertha. *Growing Your Herb Business.* Pownal, Vt.: Storey Communications, Inc., 1994.

Smith & Hawken, editors. *The Book of Outdoor Gardening.* New York: Workman Publishing Company, Inc., 1996.

Sturdivant, Lee. *Herbs for Sale: Growing and Marketing Herbs, Herbal Products and Herbal Know-How.* Friday Harbor, Wash.: San Juan Naturals, 1994.

Theiss, Barbara, and Peter Theiss. *The Family Herbal.* Rochester, Vt.: Healing Arts Press, 1993.

Tyler, Varro E. Ph.D. *The Honest Herbal.* New York: Pharmaceutical Products Press, 1993.

Wardwell, Joyce A. *The Herbal Home Remedy Book.* Pownal, Vt.: Storey Communications Inc., 1998.

Yepsen, Roger B., editor. *The Encyclopedia of Natural Insect & Disease Control.* Emmaus, Penn.: Rodale Press, 1984.

Resources

HERB SEEDS

Atlee Burpee
Warminster, PA 18974
(800) 888-1447
Web site: www.burpee.com

The Cook's Garden
PO Box 535
Londonderry, VT 05148
(800) 457-9703
Web site: www.cooksgarden.com

Gurney's Seed and Nursery Company
110 Capital Street
Yankton, SD 57079
(605) 665-1930

Harris Seeds
PO Box 22960
Rochester, NY 14692-2960
(800) 514-4441

Henry Field's Seed & Nursery Company
415 North Burnett
Shenandoah, IA 51602
(605) 665-9391

Johnny's Selected Seeds
Foss Hill Road
Albion, ME 04910-9731
e-mail: homegarden@johnnyseeds.com
(207) 437-4301

Nichols Garden Nursery
1190 North Pacific Highway
Albany, OR 97321-4580
e-mail: nichols@pacificharbor.com
(541) 928-9280
Web site: www.pacificharbor.com/nichols/

Park Seed
1 Parkton Avenue
Greenwood, SC 29647-0001
e-mail: info@parkseed.com
(800) 845-3369
Web site: www.parkseed.com

Seeds of Change
PO Box 15700
Santa Fe, NM 87506-5700
e-mail: gardener@seedsofchange.com
(888) 762-7333
Web site: www.seedsofchange.com

Shepherd's Garden Seeds
30 Irene Street
Torrington, CT 06790
(860) 482-3638
Web site: www.shepherdseeds.com
free catalog

R. H. Shumway
PO Box 1
Graniteville, SC 29829
(803) 663-9771

Territorial Seed Company
PO Box 157
Cottage Grove, OR 97424
(541) 942-9547
Web site: www.territorial-seed.com

Vermont Bean Seed Company
Garden Lane
Fair Haven, VT 05743
(803) 663-0217

HERB PLANTS

Companion Plants
7247 North Coolville Ridge
Athens, OH 45701
(740) 592-4643
Web site: www.frognet.net/companion_
    plants/
catalog, $3

PapaGeno's Herb Garden
1620 Otoe Street
Lincoln, NE 68502
e-mail: herbstogo@Prodigy.net or
papageno@navix.net
(402) 423-6179
Web site: www.papagenos.com
herb plants and seeds, and herbal products

Rasland Farm
Route #1, Box 65C
Godwin, NC 28344-9712
(910) 567-2705
Web site: www.alcasoft.com/rasland/
catalog, $3

Renaissance Acres Organic Herb Farm
4450 Valentine Road
Whitmore Lake, MI 48189
(313) 449-8336
Web site: www.apin.com/herbs/
catalog, $3

Richters Herbs
357 Highway 47
Goodwood, ON
LOC 1AO, Canada
e-mail: catalog@richters.com
(905) 640-6677
Fax: (905) 640-6641
Web site: www.richters.com
free catalog

Sandy Mush Herb Nursery
316 Surrett Cove Road
Leicester, NC 28748-5517
(828) 683-2014

Southern Perennials & Herbs
98 Bridges Road
Tylertown, MS 39667-9338
e-mail: sph@neosoft.com
(601) 684-1769
Web site: www.s-p-h.com

Well Sweep Herb Farm
205 Mount Bethel Road
Port Murray, NJ 07865
(908) 852-5390
catalog, $2

ORGANIC GARDEN SUPPLIES

Gardener's Supply Company
128 Intervale Road
Burlington, VT 05401
(800) 955-3370
Web site: www.gardeners.com

Peaceful Valley Farm Supply
PO Box 2209
Grass Valley, CA 95945
(530) 272-4769 or (888) 784-1722

GARDEN TOOLS

Earthmade Products
PO Box 609
Jasper, IN 47547-0609
(800) 843-1819
Web site: www.earthmade.com

Lee Valley Tools, Ltd.
PO Box 1780
Ogdensburg, NY 13669-6780
e-mail: customerservice@leevalley.com
(800) 871-8158
Web site: www.leevalley.com

A. M. Leonard
PO Box 816
Piqua, OH 45356
(800) 543-8955
Web site: www.amleo.com

MAGAZINES AND NEWSLETTERS
Check for newsletters in your area, too.

Herbalgram
Journal of the American Botanical Council
and the Herb Research Foundation
PO Box 201660
Austin, TX 78720
(512) 331-8868
Web site: www.herbalgram.org
e-mail: abc@herbalgram.org

The Herb Companion
PO Box 7714
Red Oak, IA 51591-0714
(800) 456-5835

Herb Gatherings:
The Newsletter for the Thymes
10949 East 200 South
Lafayette, IN 47905-9453

The Herb Quarterly
PO Box 689
San Anselmo, CA 94979-0689
e-mail: HerbQuart@aol.com
(415) 455-9540 or (800) 371-HERB
Web site: www.TheHerbQuarterly.com

Herbs for Health
PO Box 7708
Red Oak, IA 51591
(800) 456-6018

Organic Gardening
33 East Minor Street
Emmaus, PA 18098
(610) 967-5171

WEB SITES OF INTEREST

Algy's Herb Page
www.algy.com/herb

American Herbalist's Guild
www.healthy.net/herbalists/

**Frontier Natural Products Co-op
Web Site**
www.frontiercoop.com

Garden Escape Home Page
www.garden.com

The Garden Gate
www.prairienet.org/garden-gate

Henriette's Herbal Homepage
http://sunsite.unc.edu/herbmed/
goodlink.html

**Department of Horticulture,
Pennsylvania State University**
http://hortweb.cas.psu.edu

Herb Research Foundation
www.herbs.org

The Herb Society, United Kingdom
http://sunsite.unc.edu/herbmed/HerbSociety

Internet Library of Herbalism
http://herb.com/herbal.html

Organic Gardening Links
www.prairienet.org/garden-gate

The Whole Herb
www.wholeherb.com

HERB BUSINESS NETWORKS

**The Herb Growing and
Marketing Network**
Box 245
Silver Spring, PA 17575
(717) 393-3295
Web site: www.herbworld.com (herb
business information)
Web site: www.herbnet.com (general herb
information)

International Herb Association
PO Box 317
Mundelein, IL 60060-0317
(847) 949-4372
Web site: www.hcrb-pros.com
e-mail: haoffice@aol.com

OF OTHER INTEREST
*Check herb magazines and newsletters for
other herb-related interests.*

Dry Creek Herb Farm & Learning Center
13935 Dry Creek Road
Auburn, CA 95602
(530) 878-2441
classes, gift shop, gardens

The Herb Society of America
9019 Kirtland-Chardon Road
Kirtland, OH 44094
(440) 256-0514
Web site: www.herbsociety.org

Mimbres Farms
HC 15 PO Box 845
Hanover, NM 88041
(505) 536-9681
e-mail: mimbresfarms@juno.com
dried herbs for sale

Sabbathday Lake Shaker Herb Farm
707 Shaker Road
New Gloucester, ME 04260
(207) 926-4597
free catalog

United Plant Savers
PO Box 98
East Barre, VT 05649
(802) 479-9825
Web site: www.plantsavers.org
dedicated to saving wild herbs

Index

Other Storey Titles You Will Enjoy

At Home with Herbs: Inspiring Ideas for Cooking, Crafts, Decorating, and Cosmetics, by Jane Newdick. 224 pages. Hardcover. ISBN 0-88266-886-2.

The Big Book of Gardening Secrets, by Charles W. G. Smith. 352 pages. Paperback. ISBN 1-58017-017-X.

Contained Gardens: Creative Projects and Designs, by Susan Berry and Steve Bradley. 160 pages. Hardcover. ISBN 0-88266-899-4.

Easy Garden Design, by Janet Macunovich. 176 pages. Paperback. ISBN 0-88266-791-2.

Herbal Tea Gardens, by Marietta Marshall Marcin. 160 pages. Paperback. ISBN 1-58017-106-0.

Gifts for Herb Lovers: Over 50 Projects to Make and Give, by Betty Oppenheimer. 128 pages. Paperback. ISBN 0-88266-983-4.

Growing Your Herb Business, by Bertha Reppert. 192 pages. Paperback. ISBN 0-88266-612-6.

The Herb Gardener: A Guide for All Seasons, by Susan McClure. 240 pages. Paperback. ISBN 0-88266-873-0.

The Herbal Body Book: A Natural Approach to Healthier Hair, Skin, and Nails, by Stephanie Tourles. 128 pages. Paperback. ISBN 0-88266-880-3.

The Herbal Home Remedy Book: Simple Recipes for Tinctures, Teas, Salves, Tonics, and Syrups, by Joyce A. Wardwell. 176 pages. Paperback. ISBN 1-58017-016-1.

The Herbal Home Spa: Naturally Refreshing Wraps, Rubs, Lotions, Masks, Oil, and Scrubs, by Greta Breedlove. 160 pages. Paperback. ISBN 1-58017-005-6.

The Herbal Palate Cookbook, by Maggie Oster and Sal Gilbertie. 176 pages. Paperback. ISBN 1-58017-025-0.

Making Herbal Dream Pillows, by Jim Long. 64 pages. Hardcover. ISBN 1-58017-075-7.

The Pleasure of Herbs: A Month-by-Month Guide to Growing, Using, and Enjoying Herbs, by Phyllis Shaudys. 288 pages. Paperback. ISBN 0-88266-423-9.

Secrets of Plant Propagation, by Lewis Hill. 168 pages. Paperback. ISBN 0-88266-370-4.

Shaker Medicinal Herbs: A Compendium or History, Lore, and Uses, by Amy Bess Miller. 224 pages. Hardcover. ISBN 1-58017-040-4.

Sleeping with a Sunflower: A Treasury of Old-Time Gardening Lore, by Louise Riotte. 224 pages. Paperback. ISBN 0-88266-502-2.

These books and other Storey books are available at your bookstore, farm store, garden center, or directly from Storey Books, Schoolhouse Road, Pownal, Vermont 05261, or by calling 1-800-441-5700. Or visit our Web site at www.storey.com.